DATE DUE

Nurses
in the
Workplace

Nurses in the Workplace

Edited by
Marie E. Cowart
William J. Serow

SAGE PUBLICATIONS
International Educational and Professional Publisher
Newbury Park London New Delhi

For information address:

SAGE Publications, Inc.
2455 Teller Road
Newbury Park, California 91320

SAGE Publications Ltd.
6 Bonhill Street
London EC2A 4PU
United Kingdom

SAGE Publications India Pvt. Ltd.
M-32 Market
Greater Kailash I
New Delhi 110 048 India

Printed in the United States of America

Library of Congress Cataloging-in-Publication Data

Main entry under title:

Nurses in the workplace / edited by Marie E. Cowart, William J. Serow.
    p.   cm.
  Includes bibliographical references and index.
  ISBN 0-8039-4313-X (cl)
    1. Nurses—United States—Supply and demand.   2. Nurses—Florida—
Supply and demand.   3. Nurses—Employment—United States.
4. Nurses—Employment—Florida.   5. Nursing—Social aspects—United
States.   I. Cowart, Marie E.   II. Serow, William J.
    [DNLM: 1. Nursing Staff—organization & administration.
2. Personnel Management.   WY 30 N974]
RT86.73.N85   1992
331.12′91362173′0973—dc20   91-40479
                                                                      CIP

92 93 94 95 10 9 8 7 6 5 4 3 2 1

Sage Production Editor: Diane S. Foster

Contents

Foreword

The 1980s was a decade of tumultuous change in the health care system. As the largest group of health care workers, these changes had perhaps the greater impact on nurses. This book documents the status of nursing at the end of the decade with particular emphasis on problems in the state of Florida.

What have we learned from this review? First, it is clear that the factors affecting the supply and demand for nurses are complex. The factors are so complex, in fact, that we not only may have difficulty in predicting future trends but are not even certain of the gravity of the current "shortage." Questions are raised concerning the reliability of current data describing demand for nurses.

We also learn that, despite the fact that volumes have been written on techniques to recruit and retain nursing personnel, few of these techniques have been used by the major employers of nurses—hospitals and nursing homes. It also appears that few nursing education programs have formal, active recruitment efforts.

One of the important themes throughout these writings and others is that of workplace redesign. Chapter Thirteen describes some of the innovative programs being tested in Florida hospitals and the role of the nurse executive in fostering and implementing these programs. Unfortunately, it appears that such efforts are being tested in very few institutions and often meet resistance from institution management, physicians, government regulators, and others.

A second important theme is one of definition. What are the educational and/or experience requirements of a registered nurse? What about a nurse practitioner? What role should the licensed practical nurse play? While state nurse practice acts provide some definitional differences, actual workplace practice often blurs these distinctions. For example, a registered nurse may have a two-, three-, or four-education background. Starting salaries often vary only by pennies between these various levels of education. In most employment settings, there may be no differences in work assignments between registered nurses with these various educational levels despite the fact that there is a clear difference in both depth and breadth of educational preparation and potential for future growth in an organization.

Despite the fact that much change occurred in the health care system in the 1980s, it appears that more change is ahead because our health care system still suffers from fundamental problems. Once again, these changes will affect the nurse more than any other group. To move ahead, it is necessary to know where we've been. These writings provide some of those answers and are an important foundation upon which to design the future.

As we prepare for the future, a final note is appropriate. Workplace redesign and worker definition are not unique to the nursing profession. These issues are being addressed throughout the public and private sectors. Imaginative nursing leaders may find useful models outside the health care setting.

JAMES J. BRACHER

Acknowledgments

Seldom is a book such as this produced solely by the authors. This work has had much support, which we acknowledge and express our heartfelt appreciation. Initially, the convictions of James Bracher, Executive Director, and Peter Levin, Chair of the Florida Health Care Cost Containment Board, of the need to learn more about the working conditions in the various health care industries, in light of the 1987 shortage of nurses, led to the Florida Health Care Cost Containment Board's funding the research. The Florida Association of Homes for the Aged and the Florida Health Care Association of Homes gained the attention of the Florida Legislature who authorized the study. Allen Pearman, Director of Research of the Florida Health Care Cost Containment Board, and Dianne Speake, who began as Project Director for the Board and later joined the study staff as Research Associate, were both consistent in their support through the study design process and in assuring that the needed data were obtained. The technical advisory panel headed by Barbara Donoho (now Chief Executive Officer of St. Anthony's Hospital) and Peter Levin (Dean of the University of South Florida School of Public Health), which included nursing and executive officer leaders of professional associations, hospitals, nursing homes, home health and supplemental staffing agencies, and educational programs, provided input, and facilitated initial dissemination of the study results. Susan Carlson organized and interpreted the vast quantities of nursing literature that provided the basis for the design of the larger study. Countless hours were donated by the 287 hospitals, 460 nursing homes, 212 home health agencies, 29 hospices, 197 temporary staffing agencies, and 53 nursing education programs in completing the lengthy and complex questionnaires providing the data base for the research. The study staff, Winnie Schmelling, Yen Chen, Ann Shuford, and Dan Vickers, provided daily commitment to the project for months on end. Finally, our thanks go to the staff at Sage Publications, Inc., and in particular, to our editor, Christine Smedley, who envisioned the value of the project and saw the volume to completion. The content is the sole responsibility of the authors, but our thanks go to these individuals and others for their many contributions.

MARIE E. COWART
WILLIAM J. SEROW

Introduction

MARIE E. COWART

WILLIAM J. SEROW

Nursing personnel are important. In the health care system, they constitute approximately half of the employees; registered nurses, licensed practical nurses, and nursing assistants number about 3 to 4 million individuals (*Seventh Report to the President and Congress*, 1990). Much of the direct care of patients in this nation is provided by nurses. More generally, the study of nursing personnel affords the opportunity to examine a large labor force in the service industries made up largely of women.

The examination of nursing personnel at this time is particularly significant because of the dramatic changes occurring in the health care system. These changes affect the numbers and use of nurses. The issues underlying changes in the health care system and in the supply and demand for nursing personnel are complex; no simple explanations underlie the recent nursing shortage.

One contributor to fluctuations in the use of nursing personnel is the adjustment that has occurred in the health care system due to cost containment regulations and, more specifically, to the transitions that have occurred in Medicare reimbursement from retrospective payment to a prospective payment system for hospital services. This single policy change has not only affected hospitals but has triggered a ripple effect in the entire long-term care system, altering the patient mix in nursing homes, home health care, and other community-based services (Wood & Estes, 1990). Such changes have affected the numbers and functions of health care personnel, particularly nursing personnel (DeVries, 1986; *Seventh Report to the President and Congress*, 1990). The policy triggered shorter lengths of stay and increasing intensity of illness levels of patients with the effect of a changed work environment and altered roles of the nursing staff in hospitals, nursing homes, and other settings where nurses are employed. Alternative work environments in ambulatory and community settings have contributed to the demand for nurses and have provided increased employment options for nursing personnel.

Another factor affecting the demand for and use of health personnel, particularly nurses, is the aging of our population. An increasingly elderly population has fueled the increased need for nurses (Serow, Sly, & Wrigley, 1990). In particular, the fastest growing age group, those over 85 years old, with frailties, chronic conditions, and limited function, forecasts the need for expansion in all levels of long-term care services, with the accompanying increases in nursing personnel, particularly ancillary workers.

The rapid growth in technology in medical diagnosis and treatment has increased the demand for personnel, contributed to shorter lengths of stay in acute care hospitals, and altered diagnostic and treatment approaches. Increased technology has increased work loads and stimulated the growth of highly trained specialty personnel including nursing specialties. Hospitals have become critical care units with nurses making more complex and independent decisions.

Increased prevalence and incidence of AIDS, substance abuse, and related conditions not only have increased the demand for personnel but have altered working conditions for direct services personnel by increasing occupational hazards.

Such widespread changes almost assure that there will continue to be an increasing demand for nurses; yet, over time, there have been periods when nurses have been difficult to locate and recruit. Such conditions underscore the importance of gaining a better understanding of the dynamics of the workplace for nurses. Most studies about nurses draw a sample from one institution or from several similar facilities. The constant movement of nurses from employer to employer, however, calls for a fresh approach to the examination of nurses. In this study, we look critically at nurses from the perspective of employers in four industries: acute care hospitals, nursing homes, home health agencies, and hospices. Some limited information about nurses working in public health and temporary staffing agencies is also presented. This more comprehensive approach will allow for different analyses of the dynamics in the nurse labor market. The purpose of the book is to illustrate some of these dynamics and suggest how they differ across types of employers. While the data reported here pertain to the situation in the State of Florida at the end of the 1980s, there is little reason to doubt the applicability of our findings to other locations.

The book opens with an extensive review of the nursing shortage literature from 1983 to 1989. This review evaluates the literature in terms of its value in explaining the dynamics of the nurse labor force and market. This review focuses on the causes and impacts of the recent nursing shortage. We then critically examine national projections of the need for nurses in various states. Such projections, however, do not reflect the individual variations in population by state and thus do not necessarily accurately project for states with demographic qualities that differ from national norms. We also examine recent policies adopted by individual states. Because most nurses enter the pool of available nurses upon graduation from their basic nursing education program, issues related to nursing education are also addressed.

We begin our discussion of the survey of four health industries' nursing personnel with a chapter describing the political context and methodology of our study. Then, findings for hospitals, nursing homes, community-based employment, and temporary staffing agencies are presented. A thoughtful examination of the similarities and differences in these markets with regard to nursing personnel is presented and includes implications for "corporatization" and a discussion about the implications for the nurse labor market. Several further analysis chapters allow for the perspectives of a former hospital administrator, a nurse executive, and a recruitment and retention specialist. The book closes with reflections on the implications of our findings for public, institutional, and professional policymakers.

ONE

Perspectives of Nursing Personnel in the 1980s

SUSAN M. CARLSON

MARIE E. COWART

DIANNE L. SPEAKE

The recent shortage of nursing and other allied health personnel in health care institutions raises a number of important questions: What are the historical trends in the supply of and demand for nursing personnel? What impact does this shortage have on health care costs and quality of care in our hospitals and nursing homes? What are health care institutions, nursing schools, and the federal government doing to alleviate the problem? In this chapter, we examine these questions concerning the nursing shortage by reviewing and critically evaluating relevant literature recently published in professional periodicals and academic journals.

Historical Trends

Nursing shortages in the United States are not new. As early as 1920, the United States experienced a major shortage of graduate nurses (Flanagan, 1976). Just 12 years later, in the context of the Great Depression, however, the supply of graduate nurses seriously outstripped the demand for their services. The onset of World War II increased the demand for nurses to staff hospitals at home and to serve overseas on the war fronts. In response to this increased demand, new nursing schools opened, and the length of training was

shortened (Flanagan, 1976). Following the war, the demand for nursing services increased rapidly, producing another serious shortage.
The total number of nurses employed in U.S. hospitals increased by
20,000 between 1944 and 1945, and the number of student nurses
grew, yet this expansion of supply could not keep pace with explo-
sive demand. Hospital admissions rose by 220,000, and the average
daily hospital census increased by 100,000 patients during this period (Flanagan, 1976).

Early in the 1960s, the nurse vacancy rate reached an all-time high
of 23% (Aiken, 1984). The introduction of Medicare and Medicaid in
1965 caused hospital administrators to fear a nursing shortage of un-
precedented proportions. In anticipation of this increased demand for
nurses, however, Congress passed the Nurse Training Act of 1964
(Public Law 88-581) to (a) increase the quantity and quality of nurse
training programs, (b) increase the enrollment levels of disadvantaged
students, (c) increase the supply of nurses in underserved areas (i.e.,
rural and inner-city locations), and (d) upgrade the skills of existing
nurses (Eastaugh, 1985). Due to the availability of financial aid under
the Nurse Training Act, nursing school enrollments increased. In addition, trained nurses increased their labor force participation from 55%
in 1960 to 70% in 1972 in response to wage increases (Aiken, 1984).
Thus relatively low vacancy rates characterized the period immedi-
ately following the enactment of Medicare and Medicaid—a situation
that would change rapidly.

During the 1970s, nurse vacancy rates in hospitals climbed dramatically despite increased nursing school enrollments driven by the entry
of the postwar baby boom cohort (Aiken, 1984). A chronic shortage of
nurses existed until the recession of 1981-1982 and its aftermath.

In sum, the U.S. market for nurses has experienced several periods of acute and chronic shortage since the 1920s. To understand
the labor market conditions in the 1980s and the dimensions of the
current shortage crisis, we now turn to a discussion of how researchers define and measure a nursing "shortage."

Definitions and Measurement
of the Nursing Shortage

The hospital industry defines a nursing shortage in terms of the
number of budgeted, unfilled full-time equivalent (FTE) positions

for RNs. The shortage is measured by the vacancy rate—that is, the ratio of unfilled FTE positions for RNs to the total number of such budgeted positions in the unit of interest. Existing studies rely on this definition and measurement procedure to support their claims of a nursing "shortage." The literature reveals two reasons to doubt that the hospital industry definition offers an adequate account of the staffing problems that hospitals and nursing homes now face and that the vacancy rate actually measures a *shortage* of nursing personnel.

Prescott, Dennis, Creasia, and Bowen (1985) argue that the hospital industry definition of the nursing shortage only covers one potential type of staffing shortage that hospitals and other health care institutions may experience. Three other types of shortage may also affect the ability of the nursing staff to provide an adequate level of care for patients. First, a *transient shortage* may be produced when there are unanticipated staff absences and/or unpredictable changes in staffing needs. Second, there may be a *scheduling shortage* due to understaffing of certain shifts. Finally, there may be a *position shortage* due to insufficient allocation of positions and/or the wrong mix of positions—a planned and predictable form of shortage due to fiscal constraints and/or changes in the unit such as in the case mix. In sum, reliance on the vacancy shortage definition and the vacancy rate measure may lead to a serious bias in estimates of the degree of the nursing shortage experienced within a given unit.

Several authors (e.g., Aiken, 1987; Curran, Minnick, & Moss, 1987) suggest caution in interpreting the vacancy rate as a measure of nursing "shortage" because the base of the measure (i.e., the total number of budgeted positions) reflects financial constraints that hospital administrators face as well as their nursing needs. Johnson and Vaughn (1982, p. 503), however, argue more strongly against use of the vacancy rate as a measure of "shortage" (i.e., lack of supply). They contend that the vacancy rate is an attribute of the staffing script within a given hospital; it is not a measure of supply—or lack thereof—nor is it a measure of real human beings either employed or available for employment. Instead, the vacancy rate is a function of the demand for staff and the staffing structure within the hospital, not the supply of nurses in the market.

Turnover rates are measures of separations from employment in relation to the number of filled positions. Estimates of turnover rates can vary depending on whether individuals or FTEs are the basis for determining the rate of job separation. Turnover is related to employee job satisfaction as well as personal characteristics. One important component of job satisfaction is perceived control over work or autonomy (Weisman, Alexander, & Chase, 1981; Wise, 1990).

Vacancy and turnover rates are used as primary evidence in support of the claim of a current nursing "shortage." Their limitations must be kept in mind, however, when examining "shortage trends."

Nursing Shortage Trends

In 1981, the American Hospital Association (AHA) conducted the Nursing Personnel Survey. The sample for the survey consisted of 1,222 community hospitals nationwide, of which 59.9% returned questionnaires. The study used the vacancy definition of nursing shortage and compared the shortage of registered nurses (RNs), licensed practical/vocational nurses, and nurse aides/orderlies using the vacancy rate. The results showed that RNs had the highest average vacancy rates of the three categories of nursing staff—16.6% for full-time and 17.3% for part-time positions (Beyers, Mullner, Byre, & Whitehead, 1983). Nurse aides/orderlies had the lowest vacancy rates—2.7% full-time, 5.4% part-time—while licensed practical/vocational nurses fell between the two extremes—7.6% full-time, 11.8% part-time (Beyers et al., 1983, p. 27). The 1981 AHA study also showed that vacancy rates were highest in small hospitals, in investor-owned hospitals, and in the South (Beyers et al., 1983, p. 28). Finally, within hospitals, intensive/coronary care units (ICU/CCUs) had the highest vacancy rates for both full-time and part-time nursing staff—22.1% and 24.7%, respectively.

The major study cited to support the claim of a current nursing shortage in both the popular press (e.g., Clark, 1987; Lewin, 1987) and the professional and academic literatures (e.g., Aiken, 1987; Norhold, 1987) was sponsored by the American Organization of Nurse Executives (AONE) in December 1986 (Curran et al., 1987). The random sample for the study consisted of one third of the hospitals in the United States—a total of 2,316, 44% of which responded to the survey. Most claims of a nursing shortage rest upon a single piece of evidence from this study—the results showed that the vacancy rate for registered nurses had increased from the 6.3%

reported by the American Hospital Association's Nursing Personnel Study conducted in September of 1985 to 13.6% in December 1986—more than a 100% increase in a little more than one year (Curran et al., 1987, p. 444). The results also showed that more than two thirds of these RN vacancies were for full-time staff positions.

Overall, 17% of all hospitals in the AONE study reported that they had *no* vacancies for RNs compared with 35% making such reports in September 1985. In other words, more than 80% of all hospitals had RN vacancies in December 1986. By region, hospitals in the mid-Atlantic states reported the lowest range of no vacancies (4%), the west north central region the highest (31%), while the south Atlantic region fell in between with 26% (Curran et al., 1987, pp. 444-445).

In other comparisons, the AONE study showed that larger hospitals had higher vacancy rates for RNs than smaller hospitals. By ownership type, nongovernment for-profit hospitals experienced vacancy rates higher than the national average, in excess of 15%. In contrast, 27% of federal government-owned hospitals reported no RN vacancies.

In contrast to RN vacancy rate patterns, the AONE study showed that the vacancy rates for LPN/vocational nurses and nurse aides/orderlies were considerably lower—7.6% and 5.8%, respectively (Curran et al., 1987). In addition, more than 50% of the hospitals reported that they had no vacancies for LPN/vocational nurses or nurse aides/orderlies in December 1986.

The situation in Florida was similar to that of the nation as a whole. In January 1987, the Florida Health Care Association and Florida Association of Homes for the Aging jointly conducted a survey of 109 hospitals, nursing homes, and home health agencies in Hardee, Highlands, Hillsborough, Manatee, Pasco, Pinellas, and Polk counties. These health care providers reported vacancies for all nursing positions of 17% for hospitals, 14% for nursing homes, and 7% for home health agencies. Thus the vacancy rate for the hospitals in this study was higher than for the nation as a whole.

In another study, the Florida Hospital Association conducted a survey of its membership of 229 hospitals in 1987. The results obtained from 135 of its members (59%) provide a snapshot of staffing conditions during the week of May 18, 1987. During that week, there were approximately 2,348 FTE vacancies for registered nurses in Florida—a slight increase from the 2,250 vacancies in 1982. The overall vacancy rate of 10.4% was slightly lower than the 11.1% rate obtained in a similar study in 1982 and the 13.6% vacancy rate in the nation as a whole in December 1986 (Curran et al., 1987). The vacancy rate varied across regions of the state, ranging from 8% to 14%. The vacancy rate for these hospitals is lower than that for the hospitals in the Florida Health Care-Florida Association of Homes for the Aging study, probably due to the more limited regional focus of the study and seasonal differences—that is, January, during the peak demand period for hospital services by winter residents, versus mid-May, when demand for such services is curtailed.

The total number of FTE vacancies for LPNs in May 1987 was much lower than for RNs during the same period—361 for LPNs versus 2,348 for RNs—and almost 50% less than the 607 LPN vacancies reported in 1982. Overall, the vacancy rate for LPNs declined from 6.7% in 1982 to 6.1% in 1987.

The Florida Hospital Association studies show that the trend for nurse aide vacancies differed from that of both RNs and LPNs. For nurse aides, the number of vacant positions *declined* from 419 to 361 between 1982 and 1987, while the vacancy rate *increased* during the same period from 3.8 to 5.5%.

From the different trends in number of vacancies and vacancy rates across types of nursing personnel, it is possible to infer changes in the staffing patterns within hospitals. For RNs, an increase in vacant positions coupled with a decline in vacancy rates between 1982 and 1987 implies that there was a net expansion in the number of FTE positions during the period. LPNs, however, experienced a decline in both the number of vacancies *and* the vacancy rate, which indicates that employment was stagnant in this category. Finally, among nurse aides, the number of vacancies declined while the vacancy rate increased, suggesting that FTE employment opportunities declined in this category. Overall, then, these results suggest that hospitals in Florida replaced their lesser-skilled nurses with higher-skilled registered nurses during the 1982-1987 period.

Nursing School Enrollment Trends

One of the major differences between the current nurse shortage and such shortages in the past is a sharp decline in nursing school enrollments. In 1984, the total number of basic RN programs in the United States was 1,477, of which more than 50% were associate degree (A.D.) programs and 18% were diploma programs. Between 1975 and 1984, admissions and graduations from basic RN programs nationwide held fairly steady. In 1984, however, admissions of first-time nursing students fell by 4% overall and almost 11% in diploma programs. Actual enrollments of first-time nursing students in 1984 fell overall by 5.3% and 11.3% in diploma programs. In addition, enrollment of RNs in baccalaureate nursing programs increased by 6.3% in 1984 to a total of 41,112 (National League for Nursing, 1987). In 1984, men made up about 7% of admissions to basic nursing programs, while minority admissions stood at almost 13%.

In 1984, there were a total of 1,254 practical nurse programs nationwide—a 3.3% decline from 1983—and 43% of these programs were located in the South. Between August 1983 and July 1984, admissions in practical nurse programs declined by 5.8% from the previous year. Actual enrollments in practical nurse programs fell 12% between 1983 and 1984. In 1984, male admissions to practical nurse programs were 6.5%, while minorities made up 21.5% of all admissions in the same year.

With the exception of the Northeast, the number of RN admissions, enrollments, and graduations increased between 1975 and 1984, while admissions, enrollments, and graduations in practical nurse programs declined during the same period in all regions except the South. Nursing school trends in Florida follow the same pattern as in the rest of the South.

Other data show that declines in nursing school enrollments have been even greater between 1984 and 1988. Between academic years 1985-1986 and 1986-1987, enrollments in baccalaureate programs decreased by 8.5% and 10.7%, respectively ("As the Shortage Takes Its Toll," 1987, p. 529, 542; Rosenfeld, 1988a). In Florida, enrollment declines between 1983-1984 and 1986-1987 were most evident in associate degree programs, while enrollments in the one diploma program in the state remained unchanged.

Since 1988, nursing school enrollments have made a recovery. In fall 1989, an American Association of Colleges of Nursing study showed that B.S.N. schools experienced an overall increase of 2.1% over the previous fall term and a 5.9% rise in first-time nursing students, probably due to increases in nursing salaries ("Study Sees RNs Still Gripped," 1990). Similarly, a National League for Nursing study revealed that enrollments in diploma schools in fall 1989 increased 8.3% over fall 1988, B.S.N. programs 6.8%, and associate degree schools 10.6% ("Enrollments Are Rising Again," 1990). It is too early to tell whether this upward movement in enrollments will continue.

Salary Trends

Aiken has reviewed the recent history of nurse wages and their relationship to the supply of and demand for nurses in the market (Aiken, 1984; Aiken, Blendon, & Rogers, 1981). She suggests that, in the post-World War II period, nurses salaries increased by 53%, while teachers' salaries rose by 100%, and salaries in other comparable female-dominated occupations rose by 73%. In addition, nurses' wages increased most sharply in the mid-1960s when Medicare and Medicaid were adopted.

During the 1970s, nurses' real wages suffered serious erosion as average increases did not keep pace with inflation. In the latter part of the 1980s, nursing salaries increased dramatically (see e.g., Bridner, 1991; "Nurses Gained New Economic Ground," 1989; "Study Sees RNs Still Gripped," 1990). Aiken (1983) reported, however, that average monthly wages for staff nurses, in constant dollars, were $758 in 1974, $708 in 1979, and $747 in 1982. Since 1982, nurses' real wages have continued to increase; yet, by 1989, they had only regained their 1972 level (Aiken, 1991). Despite the visibility of a nursing shortage in the media, nurses' real incomes averaged only a 1.45% increase per year during the 1986-1989 period (Aiken, 1991, p. 75).

Beyers et al. (1983) collected data in 1981 from a 20% national random sample of 1,222 community hospitals. They found only minimal hourly wage differences by type of educational preparation. Although bachelor's degree nurses received higher wages, the median wage for associate degree trained nurses was only about $.10 less per hour than for those with bachelor's degree preparation. Six years of experience increased associate degree nurses' hourly wage over the median starting wage by $.90 (12.2%), diploma nurses by $.85 (11.4%), and nurses with bachelor's degrees by $.94 (12.6%). The hospitals in this study reported that they paid shift and unit differentials: with rates for weekends (20%), ICU/CCU (24%), night shift (99%), and evening shift

(99%) reported. The highest pay differentials were for night shift work. More than 80% of the hospitals provided fringe benefits, including basic health insurance (94.1%), major medical insurance (91.9%). life insurance (89.4%), maternity leave with assured reemployment (85.1%), retirement (82.3%), and tuition reimbursement (82.3%).

In Florida, annual salaries for staff nurses averaged $21,704 in 1984—$21,514 for diploma program graduates, $21,298 for associate degree nurses, $22,254 for baccalaureate nurses, and $24,391 for those with a master's degree (Postsecondary Education Planning Commission [PEPC], 1988). The average annual salary of nurses in Florida was $23,071 in 1985 and $24,414 in 1986 (Florida Department of Health and Rehabilitative Services, 1983, 1985, 1987). In the most recent study (1987), data were collected from 80% of the licensed nurses in Florida and hence include many nurses well into their careers. These Florida salaries are consistent with national average salary levels of $26,600 for critical care nurses in 1987 (VerMeulen, 1988). Thus, in Florida, as in the nation more generally, there is little monetary incentive for registered nurses to invest in higher levels of education beyond the associate's degree.

Annual salaries for other nursing positions in Florida do not vary much from those of staff nurses. Nursing administrators of hospitals or home health agencies averaged $29,164 in 1984. LPNs in 1985 averaged $14,562 annually—about two thirds of the average RN salary for the same year (PEPC, 1988).

Impact of the Nursing Shortage

Articles in the popular press and professional nursing newsletters provide accounts of the serious problems nursing shortages pose for the delivery of health care in particular acute care hospitals around the nation. These articles paint a poignant picture of the day-to-day frustrations nurses face in attempting to provide quality care for a population of increasingly older and more acutely ill patients. Nurses in understaffed units suffer extreme fatigue from long hours of overtime coupled with the stress of caring for two to three times more critically ill patients than is considered to be safe nursing practice, dissatisfaction from not being able to provide the best quality care, and, most important, constant fear and anxiety about having to make life and death decisions between patients (e.g., "As the Shortage Takes Its Toll," 1987; Clark, 1987; Gorman, 1988; Holcomb, 1988; Lewin, 1987). These articles suggest that staffing shortages around the nation lead to nurse burnout, turnover, and exit from the profession. In addition, recent strikes by nurses in New York City, Los Angeles, and Chicago were primarily over the issues of inadequate staffing and quality of care ("In All Weather," 1988; Gorman, 1988; "New Federal Commission," 1988).

Articles from the popular press and professional newsletters also describe situations where RN understaffing has become so serious that hospitals have been forced to close beds and deny patients access to care ("As the Shortage Takes Its Toll," 1987; "In All Weather," 1988; Lewin, 1987). Some hospitals have even had to curtail their emergency room services for lack of adequate staff ("More Patients," 1987).

In sum, these kinds of articles offer an initial view of some of the consequences of RN shortages in specific locations. The central theme running through all of them is that understaffing in acute care hospitals seriously threatens the quality of care and, in some, even endangers the lives of critically ill patients (Styles, 1986). A careful evaluation of nursing and academic research on the consequences of nurse understaffing will show the extent to which the claims made in the more popular and descriptive accounts based on specific cases hold more generally. It will also reveal empirical gaps that the Florida study attempts to fill.

Research on the Impact of the Nursing Shortage Within Hospitals

Our search of the literature on the recent shortage yielded three empirical studies that offer evidence for some of the consequences of the nursing shortage within hospitals described in the popular press and professional newsletter sources. It may be that the current "shortage crisis" is so new that studies conducted on the effects of nurse understaffing during the past few years have yet to be published. (Given the long turnaround time for publication in most academic journals, this is not surprising.)

In a major study funded by the Robert Wood Johnson Foundation, Prescott et al. (1985) examined nurse staffing shortages in 15 short-term general hospitals nationwide during 1981-1982. Within each hospital, they asked nurse administrators to select six patient care units from medical, surgical, pediatric, intensive care, and medical-surgical specialty areas that represented high, medium, and low vacancy and turnover rates. From each of these units, they collected questionnaire data from all staff nurses and physicians on duty during the data collection week. In addition, head nurses were asked to complete a unit profile, and three staff nurses, two physicians, the head nurse, and the nursing supervisor from each unit were interviewed using a semistructured format. They used these interview data to assess the impact of nurse understaffing on nurses, physicians, and patients.

Prescott and her colleagues found that "working short" (i.e., where there are too few or the wrong kind of staff to adequately care for the number or type of patients) changed the way nurses did their jobs. They were more rushed, had to set work priorities between jobs, and even had to decide whether or not to do certain parts of their work. Providing less than optimal care for their patients caused nurses to have negative feelings and suffer from low morale. They were " 'dissatisfied,' 'disillusioned,' 'angry,' 'discouraged,' and 'burned out' " (Prescott et al., 1985, p. 130). Working short also produced strain among coworkers.

While Prescott et al. (1985) found that many doctors in their study did not feel that their practices were affected by nurse understaffing, others did report that they had to alter their work patterns due to such shortages. Unit understaffing led some doctors to spend much more time in spelling out instructions in much more detail and leaving less decision making to the discretion of the nursing staff. In addition, physicians reported observing their patients and lab work more carefully and spending more time on nursing units to pick up the slack. In some cases, doctors were reluctant to place critically ill patients in units that suffered from chronic understaffing.

Finally, Prescott et al. (1985) assessed the impact of nurse shortages on patients. First, nurses and doctors in the study reported that, when units were understaffed, monitoring of patients' conditions decreased. As a result, many physicians were not notified soon enough about patients who were experiencing problems. In addition, patients did not receive treatments on time or as often as ordered. Psychosocial intervention and paperwork also fell behind in understaffed wards.

Second, an increase in the number of errors occurred in understaffed wards. Both doctors and nurses reported concern over the greater probability of accidents—such as patients wandering in the halls, intravenous lines becoming disconnected or infiltrated—due to insufficient monitoring of patients as well as errors in medications.

The third negative impact of understaffing on patients was a lack of continuity and poorer quality of care. Sicker patients were given priority while those with less acute illnesses were often neglected or deprived of care. Nurses were able to develop less rapport with their patients. Respondents in the study differed on the question of whether the quality of care on understaffed units was safe; some felt that it was dangerous, while others viewed the situation less negatively. Most respondents agreed, however, that care given on such wards was less than optimal.

The final impact of staffing shortages on patients was the inexpedient use of hospital facilities. Prescott et al. (1985) found that the shortage of nurses on staff at times meant that patients could not enter the ICU, while, at other times, patients were admitted to the ICU due to lack of alternative, more appropriate, adequately staffed hospital space. As a result of understaffing, patients also experienced delays in being transferred into and out of the ICU, causing some to have extended lengths of stay.

In a second article based on the same 15-hospital study, Prescott and Bowen (1987) used the questionnaire data collected from the staff nurses (N = 1,044), as well as data collected by 111 telephone interviews and 89 questionnaires from former staff nurses who had recently resigned, to examine the reasons for nurse turnover and retention. Their results show that 9% of nurses who had resigned mentioned staffing problems as one of the reasons for their resignation. In addition, those who left listed work load, staffing problems, and a lack of time with patients as the three most important factors influencing their decisions to leave. Staff nurses also listed these three factors as among the ten most inadequate characteristics of their current positions in the hospital. In sum, the results of this study furnish some indirect support for a frequent claim made in the popular and professional newsletter literature—nursing staff shortages affect nurses' decisions to resign from their hospital positions and hence lead to higher turnover rates.

In the third study, Flood and Diers (1988) examined the effect of the adequacy of nurse staffing on patient outcomes and cost in a university-affiliated, 482-bed, community hospital in the Northeast. They identified two general medical units within the hospital: one that had experienced six months of short staffing in 1986 (by the hospital's own definition) and one that had adequate staffing during the same period. Patient and staffing data for each unit were collected for three months in the middle of the shortage period. Gender and age distributions of patients in the two units were similar.

The results of this study showed that patients in the understaffed unit suffered significantly more complications than did patients in the adequately staffed unit. The most frequent complications were (a) infections, including gangrene and urinary tract infections; (b) heart conditions, including congestive heart failure and arrhythmias; and (c) gastrointestinal disorders, including hemorrhage (Flood & Diers, 1988, p. 35). The generalized infections and urinary tract infections that occurred more often in the understaffed unit are preventable with good nursing care. Flood and Diers also found that, overall, patients in the understaffed unit required higher levels of nursing care due to the higher incidence of complications. In addition, the length of stay was longer in the understaffed than in the adequately staffed unit.

Finally, based on their findings, Flood and Diers estimated that the increased length of stay in the understaffed unit cost the hospital $37,730 more than the adequately staffed unit for the study period. According to the results of this study, then, nurse staffing shortages have negative consequences both for patients in terms of increased complications and for hospital costs as increased complications produce longer lengths of stay.

Shortages of nursing personnel further affect the expenses in hospitals and other settings. For example, high turnover increases the costs associated with recruitment, hiring, orienting, and supervising new personnel. Lowered productivity, until the new employee gains experience in the position, also increases costs and interrupts continuity of care and work group stability (Weisman et al., 1981; Wise, 1990).

Hospital Strategies
for Overcoming the Nursing Shortage

In this section, we review articles that describe and evaluate strategies that hospitals and nursing homes have used to remedy the nursing shortage. These strategies fall into five categories: (a) employment recruitment, (b) use of temporary and/or foreign nurses, (c) use of auxiliary personnel, (d) increased professionalism and autonomy in the workplace, and (e) nursing school recruitment and retention.

EMPLOYEE RECRUITMENT

The results of the American Hospital Association's 1981 Nursing Personnel Survey (Beyers et al., 1983) showed that 81% of all hospitals in their sample had recruitment plans; but smaller hospitals (6 to 99 beds) were less likely, and larger hospitals (300 or more beds) were more likely, to have such a plan. Hospitals in the survey used an average of 5.5 recruitment techniques. The most frequent modes were local newspaper advertising (16.7%), recruitment at local nursing schools (15.2%), other newspaper advertising (13.5%), local job fairs (11.3%), local nursing conventions (9.3%), and recruitment at other nursing schools (9.0%).

The American Organization of Nurse Executive's 1986 survey (Curran et al., 1987) showed that 63.2% of all hospitals participated in career days at high schools and colleges to influence supply and recruitment. Hospitals focused mainly on those already in nursing school, however, and spent less effort at the high school level or below in attempting to increase interest in nursing careers among younger students. The study also showed that more than a third (37.8%) of all hospitals, and 75% of those with 400 or more beds, relied on recruitment booths at professional meetings as a strategy to attract new nurses. Other recruitment techniques used by hospitals included the following: radio and television campaigns, RN refresher courses, "finders' fees," relocation reimbursement, and billboard campaigns (Curran et al., 1987).

In a more recent survey, the National Association for Health Care Recruitment (National Association of Health Care Recruiters [NACHR], 1988) found that 70% of its member hospitals had separate budgets for recruiting nursing staff and that the average budget across hospitals rose from $153,748 in 1988 to $193,300 in 1989—a 26% increase. Virtually all hospitals surveyed used local advertising and career days to recruit nursing personnel. About 75% of these hospitals contacted new nurses by visiting nursing schools and student nurse conventions. Hospital recruiters reported using the following advertising methods: nonlocal advertising (71%), job fairs (70%), national journal advertising (66%), and career directories (65%). In addition, 35% of the hospitals indicated that they used employment agencies to assist them with recruitment efforts.

In Florida, recruitment methods used by hospitals to attract nurse applicants were much the same as elsewhere in the nation. The 1987 study by the Florida Hospital Association showed that the most frequent recruitment techniques used by hospitals included high school and/or college career days, advertising in professional periodicals, displays at conferences, and radio and/or television advertising. As for the United States as a whole, Florida hospitals reported having the most difficulty recruiting for specialty areas, with 60% having difficulty attracting ICU/CCU nurses, 28% for emergency and operating room nurses, and 21% for medical-surgical nurses.

Other articles in the literature consist of more in-depth discussions of innovative techniques hospitals have successfully used to recruit new nursing staff. In a series of articles, Stoops (1983a, 1983b) argues for use of a marketing approach for nurse recruitment so that hospitals can market themselves as employers to nurses in terms that coincide with nurses' preferences.

In another article, Sullivan and Decker (1984) discuss the results of their study of the factors that might encourage inactive nurses in St. Louis to return to the field. Their results show that 74% of the 135 respondents in their study who were not employed in nursing were considering returning. The results of regression analyses show that refresher courses, long orientation, volunteer time, and graduation in the 1960s were significantly related to considering returning to nursing. Respondents in this study also saw the following employer factors as important: proximity to home, management support of staff, orientation program, salary, being in a specialty, and feeling a part of the team.

Deets and Froebe (1984) examined how employed and nonemployed nurses ranked employment incentives. Their factor analysis results show that nonemployed nurses ranked professional recognition first, followed by conditions of employment and job autonomy; part-time nurses ranked professional recognition first, conditions of employment second, and family considerations third; and full-time nurses ranked monetary rewards first, professional recognition second, and conditions of employment third. Based on these results,

Deets and Froebe (1984) conclude that professional recognition and other working conditions are important in attracting nurses back into the labor force and that higher wages are important for job retention.

In a more recent study, Neathawk, Dubuque, and Kronk (1988) asked their sample of 416 nurses drawn from five general nonprofit hospitals in five states to list the most effective and ineffective recruitment strategies and suggestions for what could be done to make nursing a more attractive career option. Their results show that hospital nurses view special pay for difficult staff shifts, incentives for new recruits, local newspaper advertising, and special incentives for staff members who successfully recruit others as the most effective recruitment strategies. The least effective strategies included job fairs, state and national nursing journal advertising, radio advertising, and use of billboards. In terms of improving the attractiveness of nursing, Neathawk et al. (1988) report that the nurses in their sample suggested higher pay and benefits, promotion of the status and image of nursing, improving career opportunities or advancement, and increasing respect for nurses among administrators and physicians.

In results that basically agree with the Neathawk et al. (1988) study, Roberts, Minnick, Ginsberg, and Curran (1989, pp. 18-19) present the following recommendations for attracting nurses to hospital work based on their analysis of a sample of 15,000 nurses and 400 hospital administrators in six major urban areas: Hospitals should (a) offer wage differentials for evenings, nights, and weekends; (b) institute more flexible scheduling options; (c) readjust daily routines to accommodate the availability of nurses to do key tasks; (d) develop compensation policies that are responsive to the needs of individual nurses (e.g., "cafeteria" benefit plans); (e) consider creating their own nursing agencies for part-timers; (f) offer incentives for part-time nurses to increase the number of hours they work; (g) establish job classifications and a corresponding pay schedule that recognize different levels of task sophistication, professional judgment, productivity, and clinical effectiveness; and (h) consider establishing child-care programs.

Finally, Stern (1982) discusses subsidized housing as another recruitment technique that has been used successfully in the Northeast, especially New York City. He argues that provision of subsidized housing for nurses as a recruitment tool is probably most effective in cities where the supply of housing is low and the cost is high. It also may be effective in inner-city neighborhoods where nurses might see provision of safe, subsidized housing as an attractive benefit.

USE OF TEMPORARY AND/OR FOREIGN NURSES

A second strategy hospitals have used to combat nursing shortages is recruitment of foreign nurses. In 1982, an article in *Hospitals* ("Recruitment of Foreign Nurses") reported that the (then) current shortage of nurses had caused large for-profit hospital chains to pursue recruitment of nurses overseas. First, they looked to the United Kingdom and Canada as potential recruitment markets. Nurses in the United Kingdom, however, lacked course work to qualify them to sit for the State Board Test Pool Examination necessary for licensure in all but one state (Arkansas) in the United States. Canadian nurses qualified for the examination, but shortages there precluded many from seeking employment in the United States. The Philippines offered the best alternative supply of nurses, because they qualified for the licensure examination. Filipino nurses experienced a high failure rate on the examination, however. The Hospital Corporation of America (HCA) established a recruitment center in Manila to select and intensively train nurses for the State Board Examination and the Commission on Graduates of Foreign Nursing Schools Examination (also necessary for immigration for these nurses). Once the nurses passed the examinations, HCA relocated them to jobs in their chain in the United States.

In 1987, an article on foreign nurse recruitment appeared in the *American Journal of Nursing* (Naylor & Sherman, 1987) reporting that hospitals are now turning to Ireland and the Philippines to recruit nurses to combat the current shortage. U.S. hospitals must compete in these foreign markets with Australia and Middle Eastern nations, however, where nurse shortages also are acute. Data for Florida in 1981 show that most of the foreign nurse graduates in the state originally had been licensed in Asia (47.7%)—most from the Philippines (45.7%)—and, of the rest, 21.4% were from Europe (primarily Britain), 15.7% were from Canada, and 12.9% were from Central America (most from Jamaica; Cowart, 1982, p. 57).

Rather than recruiting nurses from abroad, hospitals have more typically relied on temporary or supplemental nursing service agencies or nurse registries or have established internal float pools to deal with staffing shortages. A supplemental (or temporary) nursing service is an institution that employs nurses for a set wage and hires them out to hospitals and other health care facilities to meet variable staffing requirements (Laird, 1983). Of these, supplemental nursing *agencies* do employment screening, testing, payroll deductions, and licensure monitoring and fill positions for a fee or commission. Supplemental nursing *registries* act as a referral service—the nurse works as an independent contractor and pays the registry a fee/salary percentage for employment referrals. The difference between the two, then, involves the chain of responsibility and the payment mechanism.

Both hospitals and nursing homes use supplemental nursing services to deal with nurse staffing shortages and to help balance the supply of and demand for staff in an increasingly uncertain health care market environment. Laird (1983) suggests that, for nurses, the benefits of employment with a supplemental nursing service agency include flexible schedules, higher wages, and better working conditions. On the other hand, advantages to hospitals of using supplementary service nurses include lower labor costs (i.e., payment of higher hourly wages but avoiding costs of fringe benefits and the social security match), reduction of work load for regular staff, and supervisors' avoidance of interviewing and recruiting new staff.

In their study of 160 nursing directors nationwide in the early 1980s, Prescott, Dennis, Creasia, and Bowen (1983) found that hospitals in the West used supplemental nursing services more than those in other regions of the country. Hospitals used these services for the following reasons: to fill staffing vacancies (73%), to compensate for fluctuations in patient censuses (64%), to substitute for unplanned absences (65%), and/or to provide relief for permanent staff (39%). Institutions purchased 42% of supplemental nursing services for the day shift, 33% for the evening shift, and 25% for the night shift, with most supplemental nursing services used on weekends. Orientation for supplemental nurses was required by 78% of the hospitals in the study; 95% of the hospitals evaluated the performance of supplemental nurses. Finally, supplemental nurses tended to be assigned to the same unit and patients, thus continuity of care was not necessarily jeopardized.

In Florida, a recent study (Florida Health Care Association and Florida Homes for the Aged, 1987) shows the nursing shortage and high rates of turnover have caused nursing homes to be heavy consumers of supplemental nursing services. According to this study, in November 1987, 75% of nursing homes in the sample reported having problems recruiting RNs; 65% had difficulty attracting LPNs; while 80% saw recruitment of nurses' aides as problematic. Shortages were most acute on the night and evening shifts. The nursing home industry in Florida spent an estimated $6 million dollars on overtime and temporary nursing services in 1986-1987. The salaries for temporary personnel were, on the average, twice that of regular personnel.

In a major study of temporary nursing services funded by the U.S. Department of Health and Human Services, Kehrer, Deiman, and Szapiro (1984) analyzed data collected in 1981-1982 from 809 temporary nursing service agency managers, 1,162 nurse employees of these agencies, and 469 hospital and nursing home clients of these agencies. Their research shows that, at the end of 1981, there were a total of 1,300-1,600 temporary nursing service agency offices in the United States, and 75% had only been in business since 1975. These offices were organized into 400 firms or groups—small local enterprises with two or more offices, regional companies with dozens of offices in several states, and a few large corporations with scores of offices nationwide. All but three states had such agencies. Offices were disproportionately located in California, Florida, and southern New England. In terms of ownership, 98% were private, for profit. Most temporary nursing service agencies exclusively handled health care personnel—RNs, LPNs, nurse aides, and orderlies—serving an average of eight institutional clients each—five hospitals and three nursing homes—and supplying each client with an average of 12 full-time RNs in October 1981.

Kehrer et al. (1984) also found that temporary nursing service personnel were equivalent to institutional employees in terms of education and experience: 80% of temporary nursing service agencies required experience of at least one year, but only a small minority of temporary nursing service nurses had less than three years' experience. Three quarters of temporary services nurses had been recruited from the ranks of active RNs. Registered nurses chose temporary nursing employment for the following reasons: flexible hours and workdays (84%), higher hourly wages, extra income, preference for a less than full-time permanent job, and the desire to avoid hospital politics.

In terms of work patterns, nurses in the Kehrer et al. (1984) study tended to accept work assignments from more than one agency. Most worked part-time for an average of two shifts per week. Only 36% earned $10,000 or more doing temporary nursing service work. Temporary nurses usually fill staff or charge nurse positions in hospitals and treatment/medication or charge positions in nursing homes. The shifts worked consisted mainly of weekends, evenings, and nights.

Finally, Kehrer et al. (1984) examined the personnel practices of temporary nursing service agencies and found that these agencies thoroughly screened applicants and carefully evaluated and monitored temporary nurse performance. Temporary agencies assume little responsibility for orientation of their employees to institutional policies, procedures, and plant, however; they see this as the client's responsibility.

Based on the results of their study, Kehrer et al. (1984) concluded that temporary nursing service agencies did not adversely affect the overall supply of nurses in the market—they employed only 39,138 RNs in 1980. In addition, employment of temporary nurses does not affect the quality of care provided in health care institutions.

Rather than using supplemental nursing service employees, some hospitals create their own internal "float pools" of nurses to fill staffing gaps. O'Reilly (1987) reports on some of the disadvantages of such float pools. She notes that there have been extreme cases where patients have died because a float nurse administered improper medications due to lack of knowledge of the unit, procedures, and case mix. Such cases lead to, among other things, malpractice suits. In general, use of floating leads to a lack of continuity of care, and it compromises nurses' ability to maintain professional and legal standards of care.

USE OF AUXILIARY PERSONNEL

Several articles in the recent literature discuss the use of auxiliary personnel as nurse substitutes, or "nurse extenders," to alleviate the nursing shortage. Salome (1983) describes the use of monitor technicians in the ICU to monitor electrocardiograms or free up nursing staff for more direct patient care. High school-educated nursing assistants, who were cross-trained as ward clerks, completed an approved cardiac arrythmia course to become monitor technicians. The author reports that savings of as much as 40% in labor costs could be achieved by replacing monitor nurses with monitor technicians.

In a second article that examines use of technicians as nurse substitutes in critical care settings, Olson (1983) reports that technicians were taught to set up hemodynamic pressure monitoring lines, calibrate monitors, change dressings, take vital signs, measure intake and output, assist with the patients' daily hygiene, make computer entries, and assist the nurses as needed.

Olson notes that, at first, nurses welcomed the extra help in the understaffed ICU. Problems soon arose, however, as nurses found themselves spending an increasing amount of time checking the work of the technicians. Olson (1983) concludes that, while doing more routine tasks, the nurse simultaneously provides other forms of care that cannot be provided by technicians—such as giving emotional support, teaching, explaining procedures, and making assessments that affect the outcome of care.

Flores (1987) analyzed the use of technicians in another critical context by comparing the use of operating room (OR) RNs with surgical technicians—ancillary operating room staff members who function primarily in the scrub capacity including licensed vocational nurses (LVNs) and certified and noncertified operating room technicians (ORTs)—in 211 acute care hospitals in California in 1985. She found that 94.3% of the hospitals in the sample used ORTs, LVNs, or both in their ORs, while only 12 of the hospitals exclusively employed OR RNs. All of the hospitals that used ORTs/LVNs used them in the scrub capacity and in inventory maintenance. In addition, 28 hospitals occasionally used LVNs/ORTs in the circulation capacity but only when an RN filled the scrub capacity.

More than half of hospital OR managers in the study reported difficulty in hiring RNs and lower salaries as a reason for using lesser-skilled technicians. Some OR managers, however, stated a preference for employing RNs due to their flexibility and wider knowledge base, and several stated that an all-RN OR staff was their goal. Finally, the study showed that smaller hospitals had a lower ratio of RNs to ORTs/LVNs than larger hospitals.

In the final article that deals with use of auxiliary personnel to substitute for nursing staff during nurse shortages, Lipscomb, Toth, and Wurster (1982) discuss an innovative staffing model—the Nott model—that was used at Duke University in 1969-1977 when nursing shortages threatened closure of several wards. In the Nott model, almost all of the day-to-day services on the ward were provided by personnel who had no formal nurse training. In terms of cost, Nott wards were relatively less expensive than units staffed by the nursing service at Duke. Both the average cost per patient per day/bed and average labor cost per patient per day/bed were lower on Nott wards than on nursing service units. The quality of care on Nott wards was not systematically studied; however, the six surgery residents who were questioned found staffing to be adequate on Nott wards.

INCREASED AUTONOMY AND PROFESSIONALISM IN THE WORKPLACE

Many hospitals have taken steps to change the factors that the literature suggests lead to increased job dissatisfaction, turnover, and exit from the profession among nurses. Hospital administrators assume that changing these factors will alleviate the turnover problem and its attendant costs. We discuss four interrelated categories: (a) staffing and scheduling, (b) decentralization of authority, (c) development of clinical career ladders, and (d) development of preceptorship programs.

Staffing and scheduling. According to McGillick (1983), the typical nursing schedule consists of five days on duty, two days off, with possibly every third weekend off. It is not uncommon for an evening shift to be followed by a morning shift. This type of shift work takes a toll on personal and family life as well as on physical well-being (McGillick, 1983; Rose, 1984). McGillick (1983) studied the effects of a modified work schedule on job, personal, and social satisfaction. She compared a group of 40 nurses who worked the modified schedule of three 12-hour shifts followed by four days off with a group of 40 who worked a typical schedule. Both groups worked within the same institution, had similar work conditions, and had a majority of baccalaureate-prepared nurses. Those in the modified work week group had higher scores on the Nurse Satisfaction Questionnaire in the areas of working conditions, emotional climate, compensation, and higher levels of satisfaction with their professional training than those who worked a typical schedule. Finally, the modified-workweek group had higher levels of satisfaction with their social lives. From these results, McGillick (1983) concluded that more flexible scheduling can reduce burnout, job dissatisfaction, and turnover and thus enhance retention of nurses.

Bracken, Clakin, Sanders, and Thesen (1985) developed a method to predict work load, decrease uncertainty in work load demand, and devise sets of alternative strategies to deal with changes in work load. One such strategy is "buffering"—that is, prioritizing work load and putting some work in a "buffer" to do during slack time. A second strategy is what Bracken et al. (1985) call "adaptive staffing." This strategy involves guaranteeing the staff fewer than 40 hours of work per week and 80% of all full-time fringe benefits. In this way, the need for a send-home policy and overtime are eliminated. The alternative ways to handle staff shortages/surpluses involve overtime/send-home policies or new hires/layoffs. Bracken et al. (1985) found that implementation of adaptive staffing worked best and had the highest degree of support when the staff had input into the development of the plan.

Finally, Shaheen (1985) reminds us that the goal of nursing is to provide high-quality, patient-centered care. She argues that staffing/scheduling changes should not be made unless such changes have specific goals with respect to improving patient care, have a specific time frame, and have measurable outcomes that can be operationalized in terms of quality of care. Based on these premises, Shaheen discusses what she sees as an optimal staffing solution with respect to patient-centered care. In her even-day alternating schedule model, each staff nurse works 4 days and then has 4 days off, 182 days per year. She concludes (with little empirical evidence) that such a schedule provides consistent, safe patient care on a dependable schedule.

Decentralization. Barhyte, Counte, and Christman (1987) examined the effect of decentralization of decision-making authority within nursing practice units on job attendance. They compared job attendance in four units with the typical top-down, bureaucratic decision-making structure with attendance in four others having a collegial/participatory management structure within a 936-bed tertiary care hospital in Chicago using semistructured interviews—one pretest and two posttests 3 and 6 months later.

Their results show that the experimental and control groups did not differ in the degree to which work roles were codified and structured at the time of the pretest. Over time, however, significant differences appeared between groups on this variable but not on number of sick days, absent days, or leaves of absence, although regression analyses showed that level of participation in decision making had a positive impact on job attendance.

In discussing the advantages of decentralization of decision-making authority within nursing units, Salmond (1985) notes that decentralization can promote autonomous decision making, creativity, and higher job satisfaction only when staff are prepared for it in advance. Role expectations must be clearly defined, and staff must be trained to develop decision-making skills. Salmond (1985) also observes that decentralization and participatory management are increasingly advocated for use in hospitals as a means for increasing organizational efficiency, financial solvency, and staff morale and motivation.

Development of clinical career ladders. Barhyte (1987) examined the effect of a level of practice program on the retention of staff nurses in a large tertiary health care facility in Chicago. A "clinical career ladder" or "level of practice" model evaluates and rewards nurses for clinical performance. Such a program was implemented by the Chicago hospital in 1976. Barhyte collected data via a self-administered questionnaire from a random probability sample of 10% of each of the three major levels of clinical practice. The results of the study showed a positive relationship between length of employment with the facility and the level of practice. Based on these results, the authors concluded that level of practice programs may improve nurse retention.

Preceptorship programs. A Veterans Administration Medical Center in Buffalo, New York, developed a preceptorship program to combat a chronic problem with staff turnover among newly hired employees (McLean, 1987; also see Tucker, 1987). The program begins the first working day and ends two months after licensure— about five months total—although the preceptor relationship often continues informally for about one year. The preceptor is an RN who has demonstrated clinical competence, intellectual curiosity, and effective interpersonal skills; has been on the VA staff for at least one year; and expresses a desire to serve as support/teacher to a new staff nurse. After an eight-hour training session on the role, the preceptor gradually teaches the procedures and activities to the new trainee and serves as a role model.

McLean (1987) reports that, in one year, turnover among new graduate nurses dropped from 60% to 0%. By 1986, 12 of the 19 original nurses hired in 1983, and 10 out of 10 hired in 1984, were still employed at the VA medical center. Perhaps the best indicator of the way nurses felt about the program is the fact that half of those who had been through the program expressed interest in being preceptors themselves. Although the real savings was in increased staff retention, the program cost only $1,425 per nurse. Turnover costs were estimated to be between $3,000 and $5,000 per nurse for recruitment and orientation (Hinshaw, Smeltzer, & Atwood, 1987) in addition to costs from loss of efficiency/productivity until a new staff nurse achieves average work speed.

Recently, McCloskey (1990) investigated newly employed nurses' feelings about their work. She found that nurses with low autonomy and low social integration reported low job satisfaction and work motivation, poor commitment to the organization, and less intent to stay on the job, thus reinforcing the need to use strategies for increasing autonomy and professionalism such as those reported here.

NURSING SCHOOL RECRUITMENT AND RETENTION

During the mid-1980s, there was a marked decline in nursing school enrollments. Naylor and Sherman (1987) suggest several reasons for these recent enrollment declines: a decreased pool of qualified applicants, decreased availability of scholarships and aid due to federal budget cuts, ineffective recruitment strategies, increased tuition, change in the financial situation of institutions, changes in the perception of nursing as a career, and decreased availability of qualified faculty.

Rosenfeld (1988a) argues that shrinking applicant pools have forced nursing schools to lower their admission standards and to offer remediation courses. She reports that the National League for Nursing annual survey for 1986 shows that most schools offer remedial courses in reading, math, and study skills while one third also offer courses in writing and science (Rosenfeld, 1988). Associate degree programs were the most likely to offer remedial courses (75%), while only about 50% of baccalaureate and diploma programs did so.

In terms of recruitment strategies, Rosenfeld (1988) found that 90% of all nursing programs relied on high school career counselors to recruit applicants, and 87% participated in high school career days. The National League for Nursing study shows that colleges were also exploring other recruitment strategies, such as on-site day care, listing courses in the newspaper, poster/tear off campaigns, college nights/fairs, mail campaigns with follow-up, and television and radio campaigns. In addition, most schools had one person responsible for recruitment.

Styles and Holzemer (1986) outline educational goals for the profession of nursing. First, they argue, a baccalaureate degree in nursing should be the minimum preparation for professional nursing and, second, preparation for technical nursing should be an associate's degree. Numeric goals include increasing baccalaureate-prepared nurses by 619,000 over current projections for the year 2000 and decreasing the number of technical nurses by 296,000 below current projections (Styles & Holzemer, 1986). They suggest the following strategies for achieving these goals: (a) closing non-college diploma programs, (b) merging LPN and associate degree programs, and (c) doubling the output of B.S.N. programs.

Critical Assessment of the Literature

As we have seen, there is a paucity of reliable information on the impact of nursing shortages/understaffing within hospitals and other health care institutions. Most accounts are based on what Johnson and Vaughn (1982) have described as the "reasoning from anecdotal materials" method. Stories in the popular press and professional newsletters create an awareness of some of the negative consequences of the nursing shortage on nurses, patients, and hospitals based on the situation found within selected individual hospitals. Such anecdotal accounts are not substitutes for careful empirical analyses of the problems caused by nursing staff shortages.

While the existing empirical studies in the literature generally confirm some of the purported effects of the nursing shortage within acute care hospitals that are found in the popular and professional newsletter accounts, their scope is insufficient for making generalizations about such effects nationwide. Studies by Prescott and her colleagues (Prescott & Bowen, 1987; Prescott et al., 1985) offer information on the subjective assessments of doctors and nurses concerning the impact of nurse understaffing on nurses, doctors, and patients and show that understaffing-related factors influenced nurses' decisions to resign their positions within a limited sample of 15 hospitals nationwide. The Florida study collected more systematic, quantifiable data from a larger sample of hospitals, stratified by type of ownership and size, and thus allows more rigorous and statistically reliable comparisons and generalizations.

The Flood and Diers (1988) study begins to examine the empirical effects of nurse understaffing on quality of care (i.e., patient outcomes—complications and length of stay) and hospital costs. Their research, however, examines only two units within a single hospital. The Florida project follows the lead of this study in attempting to assess the impact of nursing shortages on the quality of care—operationalized in terms of concrete patient outcomes—and on hospital costs for a larger random sample of hospitals and units within hospitals.

In this chapter, we also have reviewed studies that focus on the strategies that hospitals and other health care institutions have used to cope with the nursing shortage. Existing evidence demonstrates the effectiveness of a number of strategies in reaching certain specific goals—such as increased retention/less turnover, more successful recruitment—in particular locations. The Florida study assesses the relative cost-effectiveness of different strategies in meeting recruitment and retention goals that are consistent with quality of care criteria and in accord with professional nursing practice.

Finally, there remains doubt as to whether the current crisis is caused by a shortage in the *supply* of nurses. Instead, the current shortage may in fact be due to an excess in the *demand* for RNs by health care institutions. All of the strategies reviewed here assume that the current shortage is a supply-side problem and hence attempt to augment and stabilize the supply of nursing staff in various ways. If future research shows that the current shortage is actually a function of excess demand, then new strategies that focus on altering the staffing decisions made by hospital administrators will need to be developed and assessed.

TWO

Political Climate and Approach to Policy Analysis

MARIE E. COWART

WINIFRED H. SCHMELING

DIANNE L. SPEAKE

YEN CHEN

Knowledge of the circumstances surrounding a study helps the reader understand the rationale for the study focus and design. This chapter deals with the social-political atmosphere that existed in Florida, and to some extent nationally, at the time this study was conceived. It also deals with the legislative mandate for the study, including the establishment of a statewide advisory panel. Finally, the chapter presents the overall study design.

The Changing Political Environment

In Florida in the early 1980s, the general political atmosphere in health care targeted restraining health cost increases, assuring access to care for the medically indigent, and restricting heretofore uncontrollable costs related to medical malpractice insurance. Implementation of the federal Medicare Prospective Payment System caused concern for its yet unknown impact. The effects of competition in the health care industry were beginning to be felt, however, and members of the industry generally supported public policies that would not restrict the dynamics of the health care marketplace.

The Florida Hospital Cost Containment Board (HCCB) was established in 1979 by the Florida legislature to address health care and hospital cost increases. Again in 1985, the legislature responded to concerns about continued rising costs with the 1985 Health Care Access Act. This law not only emphasized competition but allowed for the provision of technical assistance by the HCCB as well as increased regulatory authority over hospital budget increases. One of the dilemmas presented by this increased budgetary oversight was that hospitals were penalized for increased operating expenses resulting from personnel shortages. Unfortunately, when the budgetary review process was examined, the regulatory system data base did not provide enough detail to be able to make allowances for personnel salary increases or changing staffing patterns. It was with this long-standing concern that Florida HCCB faced the acute nursing personnel shortage in 1987.

As early as 1986, hospitals expressed concern that they were having difficulty locating operating room and critical care nurses. The industry soon realized that bounties paid for locating experienced staff merely resulted in shuffling staff from one facility to another instead of correcting the problem. In 1987, the Florida Hospital Association (1987) survey of 59% (n = 135) of their member hospitals reported vacant nursing positions at 2,348, up from 2,250 in 1982. The overall vacancy rate was 10.4% (see Chapter One). At this point, the hospital industry was interested in increasing the supply of available nurses to meet the needs of a growing population in Florida. The industry concerns seemed to be that the shortage was due to increased use of health services, increased variety of positions for nurses, and increased demand for nurses because of more technology and higher acuity levels.

At the same time, the nursing homes of Florida have experienced nursing personnel recruitment problems since 1986. In a 1987 survey of half of Florida's nursing homes (n = 261), three quarters reported shortages of certified nursing assistants and registered nurses (see Chapter One). The situation in nursing homes was compounded, however, by the need to maintain minimum staffing standards for licensure as well as fixed Medicare and Medicaid reimbursement levels. Resorting to the use of temporary staff to avoid violating licensure standards cost the nursing home survey respondents more than $3.5 million dollars in 1987 (Florida Health Care Association, 1987). Thus the nursing home industry conveyed the sentiment of entrapment because of the shortage and went to the legislature in late 1987 for relief.

In January and February 1988, House and Senate committees of the Florida legislature held hearings in an attempt to try to understand specific concerns about the nursing shortage. Hospital and nursing home representatives as well as those from the nursing profession presented their views. One of the difficulties was defining the public policy implications for the nursing shortage, a dilemma created by market factors.

In these deliberations, representatives of the nursing profession clarified reasons for the shortage and provided information about nursing program enrollments to show the contrast between this problem and the shortages of previous years. The profession, through the voice of the Florida Nurses Association leadership, emphasized the need to improve working conditions as well as salaries and benefits for nurses. They emphasized the lack of attractiveness of the profession to young people, particularly young women for whom many career options were now available. While emphasizing the need for long-term solutions to enhance the future supply of nurses, they also pressed for improved working conditions.

Meanwhile, the Florida Health Care Cost Containment Board (HCCCB; renamed in 1988) had adopted a two-stage study concept that would provide information about the nursing shortage and make recommendations to revise the budgetary review process so that hospitals would not be penalized for improving the mix of personnel or for raising salaries. The Board funded and commissioned phase 1 of the proposed study, a comprehensive evaluative review of the literature that would point out areas that needed further study. With the endorsement of both the hospital and the nursing home industries, the Board submitted proposed bill language for a statewide study of the nursing shortage, its extent, causes, and impacts. The nursing home industry added a provision to study the temporary staffing agencies of the state. The Florida Nurses Association insisted on nursing input into the study. The 1988 Florida Legislature passed the bill on to the Governor for signature in June 1988.

Statutory Requirements of the Study

Florida Statutes Chapter 88-894, Section 31(1) (1988), specifically required the special study of the shortage in the supply of registered nurses in and the demand for registered nurses by hospitals, nursing homes, and other providers of health care in Florida. The study was to include the following issues:

a. the extent of the shortage as it related to different types of providers of health care and specialty nursing care;

b. the causes of the shortage, including, but not restricted to, the effects of considerations of salary, benefits, working conditions, and career development;

c. the impact of the labor shortage on the availability, quality, and costs of services provided by hospitals, nursing homes, and other providers such as physicians, home health agencies, and hospices;

d. the impact of the labor shortage on the increased use of temporary nursing pool agencies by institutional providers; the influence of this trend on the availability, quality, and costs of services provided; and the costs and benefits of potential regulation of such nursing pool agencies in light of the shortage;

e. comparisons of the extent and effects of the shortage in Florida to similar features of the experience in other states as well as to national trends;

f. the need for and the feasibility of various measures to enhance the image of the nursing profession and the recruitment of individuals into the profession, including nurse recruitment centers, human services counseling efforts directed toward students at the junior and senior high school levels, local educational outreach, and job placement programs;

g. the implications of the shortage as it related to the supply of and need for related paraprofessionals and other health care workers, such as licensed practical nurses, certified nurses' aides, and nursing assistants;

h. the feasibility of allocating loans, grants, and scholarships for the purpose of providing greater incentive for and access to the study of nursing in Florida as well as the probable effects of such efforts;

i. the desirability of demonstration projects designed to test innovative and alternative models of nursing practice, roles and responsibilities, and wage and benefit structures as well as methods for the application of successful models for the purpose of addressing causes of the shortage; and

j. the need to promote educational articulation efforts designed to facilitate the transition between different types of nursing education programs.

THE STATEWIDE ADVISORY PANEL

A major provision of the law authorizing the study was to assure that a panel representative of the nursing profession, of the hospital, nursing home, temporary staffing agency industries, and others was named to provide technical advice and oversight for the study. Initially, a nine-member panel was envisioned. Plans for the study gained much visibility in the state, however, and HCCCB staff began to receive numerous calls from associations and individuals asking to be appointed to the panel. Finally, it was agreed the composition of the panel would have representatives from these groups: the state nurses association, the state hospital association, the state association for proprietary hospitals, the state voluntary hospital association, the state association of nurse executives, baccalaureate and associate degree nursing programs, allied health programs, temporary staffing agencies, the state Commission on the Future of Nursing, proprietary and voluntary nursing home associations, the Florida Health Care Cost Containment Board, offices of the state Department of Health and Rehabilitative Services (comprehensive health planning, public health nursing, and Medicaid), the state Board of Nursing, the state Department of Education vocational health education programs, as well as a rural hospital representative. The panelists represented geographic areas of the state as well as the major industry and education sectors with an interest in the study design and outcome. Appointments were made by posing the name of potential representatives to each organization. This strategy assured ample representation by nurses—instead of succumbing to a common pitfall in nursing studies of an advisory panel with a majority of other disciplines represented. The final 21-member panel included 13 nurse leaders.

At an organizational meeting, the panelists provided input into defining the related research problems, areas to explore, and concerns from the field. Throughout the study, the panel assumed the role of reviewing and endorsing the study methodology, including instrumentation. At each stage in the study, preliminary papers and recommendations were reviewed and accepted. The cochair, a nationally recognized nurse executive, was briefed prior to each meeting and provided guidance at all stages of the study. Panelists were helpful to the study in other ways. A number of members had access to additional data or were involved in other related studies that were under way. Panelists also served as disseminators of information about the study through their respective networks. They reacted to the data collection instruments and helped to maintain statewide interest and acceptance of the study findings and recommendations. Thus the panel served a number of important roles.

The Methodology

OVERVIEW OF THE AREAS OF INQUIRY

The study included seven major components. In the following sections, the purpose of each component and the major activities necessary to achieve that purpose are reviewed.

Nursing supply estimates and projections. The major activity in this component of the study was developing projections for the supply of and demand for registered nurses in Florida during the next 30 years.

The nursing supply and demand projections were done using the methodology adopted by the U.S. Department of Health and Human Services (DHHS) and published in the *Sixth Report to the President and Congress on the Status of Health Personnel* (1988). The methodology represented the "state of the art" in terms of appropriate projection techniques for the United States as a whole as well as for individual states.

The preliminary analysis demonstrated that the methodology was significantly limited in its ability to adequately project the demand for nurses in Florida during the next 30 years, largely due to underestimation of the importance of the oldest old in the Florida population base. This conclusion was based on the knowledge that, during the 34-year projection period—1986-2020—Florida's share of the total U.S. population is forecast to rise from the estimated level of 4.8% to some 6.8%, an estimated increase of nearly 70% from 11.7 to 19.7 million. For the entire country, the estimated population increase is a comparatively low 21%. Of the total population increase, some 8 million (16%) of the increase is forecast to occur in Florida. In addition, by the end of the projection period, more than one fourth (25.6%) of Florida's population will be at least 65 years of age. Furthermore, the oldest-old population, aged 85 and over, will rise by 299%, from 171,000 to 683,000. Because the elderly use health services at a far greater rate than the general population, it seemed very likely that the demand-side projections for nurses underestimated the requirements in Florida because the BHP methodology did not take these dramatic population growth and composition changes into account. For this reason, the HCCCB authorized a special substudy to develop projections that more accurately reflected the demand for nurses given Florida's rapid population growth, unique population mix (the elderly, particularly the oldest old), and the high incidence and prevalence of social conditions requiring health care (AIDS and substance abuse).

Activities in this component of the study included reviewing the literature, identifying major projection models for nursing and allied health professionals, evaluating each model, selecting key components and variables, developing a projection model for Florida, and preparing a report describing the model and documenting the projections. This evaluation and revised projection model are reported in Chapter 4.

National trends and state comparisons. This component of the study, in the form of a background paper, compared Florida's nursing shortage experience with that of other states and with the nation as a whole. Study activities included updating the literature review completed earlier and gathering information from a number of other states on the extent and impact of the shortage, available projections of supply and demand, and public and private sector responses to the shortage.

To compare Florida's experience with that of other states as well as with the national nursing shortage experience, seven states were selected: North Carolina, Nebraska, New Jersey, Maryland, Pennsylvania, Tennessee, and Texas. All of these states had published reports with lengthy lists of recommendations addressing the nursing shortage.

In general, these reports were based on public hearings and included public policy recommendations regarding licensure and nurse practice acts, regulation and certification of nursing assistants, establishment of state nursing data bases, increasing minority access to nursing education, funding of educational programs, funding for nursing scholarships and financial aid, establishment of nursing research centers, and reimbursement for nursing services.

Recommendations for consideration by the private sector included improving use and autonomy, increasing educational funding, supporting nursing research, and providing innovative and flexible benefit packages. A summary of this phase of the study is reported in Chapter 3.

Nursing education and financial support. This component of the study looked at the feasibility of allocating loans, grants, and scholarships; estimated their effect on the shortage; and explored the need for promoting educational articulation to facilitate the transition between different types of nursing programs.

Study activities included gathering and analyzing existing Florida-specific data as well as collecting information from all schools of nursing in the state on the issues of educational articulation and finance. An instrument was designed to gather the following data from all schools of nursing: trends in applications, enrollment, attrition, graduation, and qualifications of students; articulation and career ladder opportunities; financial aid; flexibility of course scheduling; recruitment and retention of students; faculty availability; faculty salaries; and concerns of deans and directors.

The questionnaire was sent to all nursing education programs, including 5 graduate, 11 B.S.N., 1 diploma, 18 associate degree, and 24 LPN programs. Programs offering certificates for nurse anesthetists and for nurse practitioners were not included in the study. The findings of this part of the study are reported in Chapter 5.

Extent, causes, and impact. The purpose of this component of the study was to examine the extent of the nursing shortage by provider of care and specialty of nursing; causes of the shortage, including compensation, working conditions, and career opportunities; impact of the shortage on the availability, quality, and cost of services provided by hospitals, nursing homes, home health agencies, and hospices; use of temporary agencies and the influence of that use on the availability, cost, and quality of services as well as the potential benefits of regulation of the temporary agency industry; and the implications of the shortage with regard to the supply of and need for other health care workers such as licensed practical nurses, certified nurse aides, and nursing assistants.

Study activities focused on the primary data collection efforts that were necessary to address extent, causes, and impact of the nursing shortage as well as the other issues specified above.

The first step was to think through each of the statutory issues and determine:

- What is the question to be answered?
- What data are necessary to answer that question?
- Are those data available?
- If so, what are the limitations of the data?

It was learned that, although a good deal of data were available, there were no comparable data across providers that would allow reasonably careful analysis of extent, causes, and impact.

Adequate data about the supply were available from the Board of Nursing, at least with regard to registered nurses (RN) and licensed practical nurses (LPN). The Board of Nursing had sent a questionnaire every two years—to RNs since 1981 and to LPNs since 1983—when licenses were renewed. The data from the RN survey have been analyzed by state staff in the Office of Comprehensive Health Planning since 1981. The data for this study were designed to complement the existing data on the supply of registered and practical nurses.

Primary data collection instruments were then designed to include the following areas of information:

- Nurse supply vacancies and turnover by classification and specialty
- Nurse supply, by classification and average daily census, during the past 5 years
- Seriousness of shortage by nursing specialty, position, season, day of week, and shift
- Staffing standards
- Staff mix by classification of age, education, and length of employment
- Affiliations with schools of nursing
- Salary information (minimum sta.ting, maximum starting, average, maximum hourly rates, and percentage at maximum) by classification, changes in salary scales, premiums paid, and availability of clinical career ladders
- Benefit information by classification
- Job content information, including percentage of time in various activities, mode of nursing practice, and changes in mode of practice
- Impact in terms of interruptions in service, overtime and recruitment expense, and quality of care

- Use of temporary agencies by classification, average expense, range of fees, and total expenditures
- Changes in staff mix and substitution strategies
- Opinions on the effectiveness of various recruitment and retention strategies

SURVEY METHODS

The Florida Nursing Shortage Study was designed to include all of the elements specified in the statute authorizing the original study extensions. Time frames were established to meet statutory deadlines as well as to provide necessary information at critical points in the legislative process. Background papers were completed prior to the survey phase. Primary data collection was planned to provide advance notification of the week for which data would be requested. It was also important that the data collection week did not fall during holiday periods or other times that might be grossly atypical.

The backgrounds of the two principal investigators included economics and nursing. In addition, two nurses with doctoral preparation were added to the study team. A graduate student with a background in demography provided much of the supervision of data entry and conducted the computer data analysis.

Sample. Names and addresses of all nursing homes and hospitals licensed by the State of Florida that report to the Health Care Cost Containment Board (HCCCB) were obtained from the HCCCB files. Federal hospitals located in Florida and nursing homes associated with Life Care programs were excluded from this study because they were excluded from the regulatory authority of the HCCCB. Names and addresses of home health agencies and hospices were obtained from the Office of Licensure and Certification (OLC) of the Department of Health and Rehabilitative Services. A total of 1,351 questionnaires were distributed by certified mail in February 1989 to the population of Florida hospitals (n = 301), nursing homes (n = 474), home health agencies (n = 544), and hospices (n = 32). Questionnaires were initially returned by 228 hospitals, 409 nursing homes, 288 home health agencies, and 13 hospices. Reminder notices were sent to all facilities, which resulted in responses from an additional 59 hospitals, 51 nursing homes, 125 home health agencies, and 16 hospices. Questionnaires to 46 home health agencies and 2 hospices were undeliverable (i.e., incorrect addresses or out of business, and one additional hospice had combined with a home health agency and was counted as part of that home health agency). Of those returned, 200 home health agency questionnaires were incomplete and unusable. Sixty home health agencies were excluded from the study because they did not provide services in the home during the week of the study, December 5-11, 1989. An additional seven agencies opened for business after the December 11, 1988, date. A total of 287 hospitals, 460 nursing homes, 212 home health agencies, and 29 hospices were included in the final sample for data analysis. Corrected response rates with one mailed reminder were very high—hospitals 97%, nursing homes 97%, home health agencies 48%, and hospices 100%—because of the statutory authority of the HCCCB to impose administrative penalties on nonrespondents.

LIMITATIONS OF THE STUDY

Several limitations of the study should be noted:

1. The data were retrieved by a variety of personnel. There was no way to control who completed the questionnaire forms. Both the chief executive officer and the chief nursing officer were required to sign the cover page, indicating that the data contained in the questionnaire were accurate and were taken from the institution's records. In some instances, business office personnel completed the budgetary information.

2. Many large hospitals and nursing homes had computerized data but many smaller agencies had to retrieve the requested data by hand. In addition, some requested data were not manually retrievable from the records of some institutions.

3. Only those home health agencies providing intermittent nursing services in the home were surveyed. Those agencies providing only staffing services did not complete questionnaires ($n = 60$). An additional 25 home health agencies did not respond to the questionnaire.

4. The sample does not include federal hospitals located in Florida or nursing homes associated with continuing care retirement communities.

5. Because the data collection is industry based, the study does not provide detailed information about the characteristics and perceptions of the nurses working for these providers of health services.

DATA ANALYSIS

Data analysis was directed at examining relationships that further illuminated the shortage of nurses in Florida's hospitals, nursing homes, home health agencies, and hospices. Employment data from each institution were used to measure the association between measured shortage and turnover in light of variation among employing institutions. More specifically, measures of shortage, (nurse-patient ratios and vacancy rates) and turnover (terminations divided by budgeted positions) were examined using measures of central tendency, correlation, ANOVA, and simple and multiple regression estimates of the effect on the "outcome" (dependent) measures of variation in "predictor" (independent) variables such as the following.

- wage and salary levels
- presence and extent of shift differentials
- type and level of fringe benefits (such as vacation and holiday leave, sick leave, and retirement programs)
- type and level of mechanism for professional advancement (such as opportunities for additional professional training, career advancement, and paid travel for attendance at professional meetings)

Temporary staffing agencies. This portion of the study was requested by the Florida legislature to improve the information base with regard to temporary staffing agencies as related to providing health care personnel. The impact of temporary staffing agencies on the operating expenses of hospitals and nursing homes had generated significant pressure for regulation during the 1988 and 1989 legislative sessions. Although the initial survey requested a great deal of information from hospitals, nursing homes, home health agencies, and hospices with regard to agency use, there were no data available from the temporary staffing agencies themselves. Thus data were collected from temporary staffing agencies 12 months after the survey of other sectors of the health care industry.

This component of the study included reviewing the literature, developing a mailing list of agencies to be surveyed, and designing and pretesting the survey instrument. The survey instrument was designed to gather the following information: ownership; services; costs; charges; orientation procedures; users of services; supervision of employees; evaluation of employees; criteria for hiring, recruitment, and retention of personnel; and length of assignments.

Because temporary staffing is a relatively new industry in health care, without a formal representative organization, a list of agencies was developed from several sources: agencies known to the HCCCB and the Bureau of Business Regulation as well as telephone listings from the 15 largest cities in Florida. Agencies were sent questionnaires and an explanatory cover letter by certified mail using the regulatory authority of the HCCCB. Subsequent to preliminary data analysis, respondents were contacted by telephone interview to complete and clarify answers. The findings for this portion of the survey are reported in Chapter 9.

Summary

While the need for this study was originally conceived in 1985, the onset of the nursing shortage two years later served to stimulate the hospital and nursing home industries, the nursing associations, and the Florida Health Care Cost Containment Board to request the Florida legislature to "do something." This study was conducted in three phases: the original review of the literature; then, building on a set of background papers, data collection from Florida nursing education programs, hospitals, nursing homes, and home health agencies, and further data collected from Florida temporary staffing agencies; and development of a Florida-specific nursing supply projection for the future. The study, conducted during an 18-month period, received advice from a statewide advisory panel including nurse leaders from a variety of organizations and settings. One of the most extensive studies of this period, it is projected to affect the general understanding of the employment conditions of nurses in four health industries in Florida.

THREE

State Policies and Legislation

DIANNE L. SPEAKE

A flurry of studies were mandated by state legislatures during 1988 and 1989 to answer questions and concerns about the nursing short-age in the United States. This chapter will highlight the nursing shortage studies from seven states and will compare the findings and recommendations from these studies with the Florida nursing shortage study. The states chosen for comparison (Maryland, Tennessee, North Carolina, Texas, Pennsylvania, New Jersey, and Nebraska) were selected because the size of their health care delivery system (e.g., in terms of number of hospital and nursing home beds per population and the number of physicians per population) is comparable to that of Florida and because these states published reports that allow for data comparison.

All studies reviewed, excluding Texas, were authorized by state legislative action; the professional nursing organizations in Texas initiated their study without legislative mandate. All studies, excluding Florida, used a commission format to study secondary data and conduct public hearings. Several of the states, including Pennsylvania and North Carolina, had state legislators on the study commission. The Florida study, in comparison, consisted of a technical advisory panel (TAP) appointed by a state agency, the Health Care Cost Containment Board (HCCCB). The 21-member TAP consisted of nursing leaders from educational institutions, professional nursing organizations, the Florida Board of Nursing, and health care organizations. Nonnurse representatives from state health agencies, health care institutions, and health associations were also included in the TAP to assure representation for both consumers and providers of nursing. All members brought unique perspectives and expertise to the TAP.

The scope of nursing data included in the state reports varied remarkably and thus limited data comparison somewhat. Most of the states did report 1987-1988 data in their reports so that data from the same time period are compared. Unlike the other states, however, the Florida study collected primary data from hospitals, nursing homes, home health agencies, and hospices. In addition, secondary data obtained from the Florida Board of Nursing, the Florida Department of Education, and health care professional associations were used to enhance the report and prevent duplication of effort.

Nursing Trends

SUPPLY OF RNs

According to the Florida State Board of Nursing, 96,185 registered nurses were licensed and residing in Florida as of May 12, 1987. Of the 96,185 RNs, 78.2% (75,248) were practicing nursing, with 59,022 employed full-time and 16,226 part-time. Of the 25,735 licensed practical nurses in Florida, 62.8% were practicing nursing. These percentages are in keeping with national statistics, which indicate there were 1.9 million registered nurses in 1984, 79% of whom were working in nursing, and 781,506 licensed practical nurses, 69% of whom were working in nursing (Richman, 1987). Florida's percentage of employed RNs is higher than that in reported statistics from Texas (77.9%) and Maryland (70%) but lower than Tennessee (98.5%), Nebraska (90%), and North Carolina (80%).

The number of Florida licensed nurses endorsed from other states is almost twice that of new graduates from Florida nursing education programs, a practice that makes Florida a debtor to other states. Unlike Pennsylvania and Texas, however, the number of nurses entering Florida by endorsement and examination continues to exceed the number of nurses moving out of the state, with an overall net gain of 57% between 1976 and 1986.

EDUCATIONAL PROFILE OF RNs

Of the registered nurses in Florida, 26.2% (19,475) hold a baccalaureate degree, 33.4% (24,844) a diploma, and 34.0% (25,254) an associate degree. There are 413 (0.6%) nurses with doctorates and

4,308 (5.8%) with master's degrees in Florida (Florida Department of Health and Rehabilitative Services [DHRS], 1987). Compared with Tennessee, Florida has a much smaller proportion of registered nurses prepared at the baccalaureate and graduate levels. Only 17.7% of the new RNs were graduates of B.S.N. programs in Florida while 82.3% were graduates of associate and diploma programs. This compares with Texas figures of 45% and 53%, respectively. National statistics from 1984 indicate 25.5% of nurses have baccalaureate, 45.3% diploma, 22.8% associate, 0.3% doctoral, and 5.6% master's degrees.

The number of graduates from nursing education programs in Florida declined 14% between 1985 and 1987. This compares with the national trend of 18.7% (Rosenfeld, 1988). Maryland experienced a 21% decrease in enrollment between 1985 and 1987 with North Carolina reporting a 22% decline and New Jersey a 18.2% decrease. Graduations declined by 17% in Florida as compared with 18% in Maryland, 55% in Nebraska, and 2.9% in New Jersey.

PRACTICE AREAS OF RNs

Of the registered nurses employed in Florida, 65.6% (44,659) practice in hospitals, 5.5% (3,714) in nursing homes, 5.7% (3,845) in physicians' offices, and 6.1% (4,120) in home health agencies. The remainder are employed in government and industry (DHRS, 1987). These figures are consistent with RN practice areas in North Carolina (66%) but are lower than reports from Texas (71.2%) and Nebraska (69%). National data indicate that approximately two thirds of the employed nurses practice in hospitals (American Nurses Association [ANA], 1985).

PRACTICE AREAS OF LPNs

Of the 25,735 LPNs practicing in Florida, 41.8% (8,460) practice in hospitals, 21.4% (4,388) in nursing homes, 11.6% (2,342) in physicians' offices, and 7.5% (1,520) in home health agencies (DHRS, 1987). At the national level, 57.6% of LPNs are employed in hospitals, 22.5% in nursing homes, and 9.1% in physicians' offices. The remainder work in private duty and various community-based settings (ANA, 1985). Both Nebraska and Texas reported higher percentages (52% and 49.8%) of LPNs employed by hospitals. The percentage of LPNs in Florida who work in nursing homes and physicians' offices is similar to that of Texas (21.5% and 12.1%, respectively) but lower than that of Nebraska (26% and 7.5%).

NUMBER OF RNs WHO LEAVE THE WORK FORCE

Each year, a number of nurses leave nursing for personal reasons including relocation, low salaries, heavy work load, lack of child care, shift rotations, and return to school (Hay Group, 1988). Currently, 5.6% (5,388) of Florida RNs are working outside of nursing and 9.4% (9,046) are unemployed. Of these unemployed nurses, 1,444 are seeking nursing employment and 7,602 are not (DHRS, 1987). These figures represent only those nurses who hold active licenses, not those with inactive licenses.

NURSE VACANCY AND TURNOVER RATES

Reports from various organizations indicated that 75% of nursing homes and 84% of Florida hospitals experienced an overall shortage of staff RNs in 1988. The majority of hospitals (57.3%) reported that the shortage was of moderate severity. The hospital RN vacancy rate in May 1988 was 15.8% compared with a 10.4% rate in May 1987 (Florida Hospital Association [FHA], 1988). Nationally, an average of 11.3% of hospital positions for RNs and 6.2% for LPNs were vacant in December 1987 (American Hospital Association [AHA], 1988). Of the states reviewed, only New Jersey had a higher RN hospital vacancy rate (17%) than Florida.

The RN FTE turnover rate in Florida hospitals decreased from a 1987 rate of 21.3% to a rate of 16.1% (FHA, 1988). The national turnover rate for RNs in hospitals remained at 20% in 1988 but the cost of each newly hired RN rose 32% to an average of $1,899 (National Association of Health Care Recruiters [NAHCR], 1988). Of the hospitals in Florida, 20% indicate the average annual (per hospital) total cost of nurse recruitment is $106,800 (FHA, 1988).

Recommendations

Of the states reviewed, all have submitted reports with lengthy lists of recommendations. Some of these recommendations are directed at public policy but many are intended for the private sector (see Chapter 2). A condensed list of state recommendations is provided in Tables 3.1 to 3.8.

The recommendations for the states included in this chapter largely focus on improving nursing image, increasing financial support for nursing education, and increasing educational opportunities. Only one state, Maryland, urged health care facilities to provide sufficient ancillary support staff to complete nonnursing tasks, one key element in work redesign efforts.

Rather than developing an exhaustive set of recommendations about the nursing shortage, the Florida study elected to make one long-term recommendation and five short-term recommendations that emphasize the need to redesign patient care to meet the current and future demands and supply of health personnel. The recommendations aim to monitor and assist providers in the redesign of organizational structures to improve and coordinate patient care.

TABLE 3.1 New Jersey: Executive Order No. 179

Purpose, Method, and Findings	*Recommendations (partial list)*

Purpose of study:
(a) Evaluate the adequacy of the current and future supply of RNs and ancillary nursing personnel
(b) Make recommendations to ensure that the supply of RNs and ancillary nursing personnel will be consistent with the health care needs of the people of this state
 	
Method:
A nursing shortage study commission consisting of 13 members was appointed. Hearings were conducted.
Findings:
Vacancy rates—
  hospitals
    RNs—5.3% in 1986; 17.0% in 1987
    LPNs—4.8% in 1986; 11.4% in 1987
  nursing homes (1987)
  180 responding homes reported 832 RN and LPN vacancies
Educational enrollments (1984-1987)—
  RNs decreased 18.2%
  LPNs decreased 6.9%
Educational graduations (1984-1987)—
  RNs decreased 2.9%
  LPNs decreased 22.2%
	1. Agencies collecting nursing health professions data should ensure the accuracy, timeliness, and comprehensiveness of data.
	2. The cost of nursing care should be determined and categorized based on patients' needs and nursing services provided as soon as feasible.
	3. Establish staffing levels that provide safe and therapeutic nursing care. Patients' needs should be identified with acuity measures.
	4. Nursing work loads should be structured to minimize performing nonnursing functions by using more support personnel and computerized clinical and management systems.
	5. Benefit options for the care of dependent adults and children should be made available to nursing personnel.
	6. Clinical nursing research should be fostered and research protocols that involve nurses should be established and/or approved by nurses.
	7. Nurse executives should have parity of positioning and reporting relationships with other senior executives in the organization.
	8. Establish a fund to assist employees to develop professional practice models to promote the recruitment and retention of nurses.
	9. Enhance positions through organizational change, participative management, and shared governance within health care settings.
	10. Begin preceptor programs for new graduates to encourage them to develop positive relations with experienced nurses.
	11. Increments in salary and status should be tied to criteria for assessing professional growth.
	12. Establish scholarship and loan programs for nursing students including minorities and the economically disadvantaged. Fund nursing program innovations in educational accessibility.
	13. Health care employers should provide financial assistance and flexible scheduling for nursing staff to continue their education.

14. The state government and private industry should accelerate a major media campaign to promote the nursing career.
15. The Board of Nursing should create a task force for planning an orderly transition to two categories of nursing by the year 2000.
16. Externship/internship and preceptorship programs should be developed cooperatively between academic and service institutions/agencies.

SOURCE: New Jersey State Nursing Shortage Study Commission (1988).

TABLE 3.2 Florida: Authorized by Florida Laws Chapter 88-394

Purpose, Method, and Findings	Recommendations

Purpose:
To study the shortage of registered nurses in hospitals, nursing homes, and other providers of health care including
(a) extent of shortage as it relates to different providers of health care and specialties of nursing care
(b) causes of the shortage including considerations of salary, benefits, working conditions, and career development
(c) impact on the availability, quality, and costs of services provided by hospitals, nursing homes, and other providers
(d) impact of the labor shortage on the increased use of temporary nursing pool agencies
(e) comparisons of extent and effects with those of other states and national trends
(f) need for various measures to enhance the image of the nursing profession and the recruitment of individuals into the profession
(g) implications of the shortage on the supply and need for related paraprofessionals
(h) feasibility of allocating loans, grants, and scholarships
(i) the desirability of demonstration projects to test innovative and alternative models of nursing practice, roles, and responsibilities, and wage and benefits structures
 	
Method:
A 21-member Technical Advisory Panel was formed and data were collected from all hospitals, nursing homes, home health agencies, and hospices.
 	
Findings:
Supply (1987)—
RNs 96,185
LPNs 25,735
Work setting (1987)—
RNs 65.6% in hospitals   LPNs 41.8% in hospitals
5.5% in nursing homes   21.4% in nursing homes
	1. The demand for and supply of those who do the work of patient care must be realigned in the various health care settings, particularly hospitals and nursing homes. This will mean, on the demand side, health care organizational restructuring and altering of the worker environment to redesign the work of patient care. On the supply side, it will require creative efforts to produce the necessary numbers and types of workers.
	2. Provisions should be made for projects in hospitals and nursing homes to define the realigned work skills of patient care needed to achieve quality outcomes. Projects should include evaluation of project implementation and wide dissemination of the results.
	3. The health care industries will need to alter the workplace to reduce personnel turnover and related expenses by addressing job satisfaction including career advancement and salary and benefit levels across all sectors of the health system starting with those most out of line.
	4. The nursing profession will need to assume responsibility for supporting the work environment in recruitment and retention of nurses through innovative practice models, image enhancement, career information, and other measures.
	5. Industrywide data collection and analysis are needed at regular intervals to measure shifts in the use of nursing and other health personnel as patient care work restructuring occurs to monitor progress and plan for the future.
	6. A coordinated nursing education system is needed to ensure student learning about patient care within the context of the total patient experience and the realities of the work setting:
	  —develop partnerships between educational institutions and hospitals and nursing homes for preparing and retraining of personnel
	  —expand state matching fund contributions to universities as well as community colleges

5.7% in doctors' offices
6.1% in home health

11.6% in doctors' offices
7.5% in home health

Employment status (1987)—
78.2% RNs employed in nursing;
78% full-time, 22% part-time
62.8% of LPNs employed in nursing;
72% full-time, 28% part-time

Nursing staff per 100 patients (1988)—
hospitals 102.5 RN
30.8 LPN
32.9 NA
nursing homes 6.4 RN
10.9 LPN
34.8 NA

Vacancy rates (1988)—
hospitals 17.2 RN
19.9 LPN
18.1 NA
nursing homes 24.7 RN
17.7 LPN
12.4 NA
home health 31.2 RN
83.3 LPN
44.5 NA

Turnover rates (1988)—
hospitals 28.3 RN
33.1 LPN
37.0 NA
nursing homes 74.1 RN
69.1 LPN
113.5 NA
home health 51.9 RN
29.9 LPN
67.4 NA

RN educational profile (1987)—
26.2% BS degree
33.4% diploma
34.0% associate degree
5.8% master's degree
0.6% doctorate

Beginning hourly salary (1988)—
hospitals RN-AA $10.31
diploma 10.43
BS 10.60
LPN 7.20
nursing homes RN-AA $9.96
diploma 9.95
BS 10.11
LPN 7.86

—increase number of baccalaureate- and graduate-prepared nurses
—promote access for nontraditional students
—phase in a minimum of a high school diploma for all categories of health personnel

Purpose, Method, and Findings, continued

Educational programs—
RNs 26 associate degree, 1 diploma
11 baccalaureate, 6 master's, 2 doctoral
LPNs 42 programs
Educational enrollments and graduations:
34% decline in RN enrollments 1983-1987
17% decline in graduates 1983-1987
Licensure data (1987-1988)—
new licenses (total) 13,004
RN by exam 3,220
RN by endorsement 6,522
LPN by exam 1,550
LPN by endorsement 1,712

SOURCE: Florida Health Care Cost Containment Board (1990).

TABLE 3.3 Maryland: SJR 27 and HJR 53

Purpose, Method, and Findings	*Recommendations (partial listing)*
Purpose: (a) Examine causes of the crisis in nursing in Maryland including the working conditions and hours (b) Examine ability of hospitals and health care facilities to remain competitive with respect to salaries (c) Examine the impact of closing hospital-based nursing schools (d) Develop incentives for retention of nurses (e) Develop recommendations for the secondary school system to encourage nursing as a career **Method:** A governor's task force to study the crisis in nursing was formed and hearings were conducted. **Findings:** Supply (January, 1988)— Approximately 50,000 RNs and 8,000 LPNs are licensed in Maryland. Employment status— Nearly 70% of the RNs in Maryland are employed in nursing; 34% of RNs work part-time. Vacancy rates— Hospital vacancy rates for RNs were 6% in 1983, 11% in 1986, and 13.1% in 1987. Turnover rates— Turnover rates for RNs in Maryland hospitals have increased from 17.8% in 1984 to 23.1% in 1986. The cost of turnover is estimated to be as high as $6,000–$7,000 per nurse.	1. Direct the Health Services Cost Review Commission to establish the hospital workers' (third-level) index for adjusting the wage and salary inflation factor effective January 1988 and a Nursing Wage Index by January 1989 to accommodate appropriate nursing salary adjustments in the future. 2. Encourage the Maryland Medical Assistance Program to allow an equal rate increase in nursing home reimbursement for long-term care facilities to be competitive. 3. Develop methods to identify nursing services on patients' bills (effective 1990). 4. Extend existing nursing transition courses to 1994 and expand sites beyond the metropolitan areas. 5. Allocate sufficient funds to permit the Maryland Board of Nursing to establish an adequate data collection, management, and reporting system. 6. Review regulations for day-care centers that inhibit the ability of health care facilities to provide day-care services. 7. Request schools of nursing to explore ways to provide curricular flexibility and alternative scheduling of nursing education programs as a means to recruit and retain nursing students. 8. Urge B.S.N programs to include courses in economic and fiscal management to prepare nurses for first-line management positions.

Educational programs—

Total enrollments in schools for RNs decreased by 21% and total graduations decreased by 18% from 1985 to 1987.

9. Encourage health care facilities to foster collaborative practice between nurses and physicians and provide sufficient ancillary support staff to complete nonnursing tasks.

10. Support efforts of professional nursing organizations in the state to educate the public about the values and contributions of nurses and nursing including the development of a statewide media campaign to promote nursing as a career.

11. Direct the Secretary of the Department of Health and Mental Hygiene to establish a mechanism to monitor the status of nursing in Maryland, reporting to the governor at least annually.

SOURCE: *Maryland Crisis in Nursing* (1989).

TABLE 3.4 Texas

Purpose, Method, and Findings	*Recommendations*
Purpose: 　To coordinate pertinent information on the shortage to allow the best decision making for Texas and its health delivery system Method: 　Review of secondary data Findings: 　Supply— 　111,500 RNs licensed in 1988; 　35% increase since 1980 　71,571 LVNs licensed in 1988; 　20% increase since 1980 　Ratio of 1 RN per 228 population in 1988 　Work setting— 　RN Employment in 1987 was 　71.2% in hospitals 　2.7% in nursing homes 　8.7% in community health 　5.8% in MD Offices 　2.3% in schools of nursing 　1.3% private duty 　7.4% other 　LVN employment in 1988 was 　49.8% in hospitals 　21.5% in nursing homes 　12.1% in doctors' offices 　2.9% in community health 　7.4% in private duty 　6.4% in other Employment status— 　64.6% RNs work full-time in nursing, 13.3% RNs work part-time in nursing, 3.8% RNs work in other fields, 67.8% LVNs work full-time in nursing	1. Increase the number of graduates from Texas generic schools of professional nursing by 50% over 1987-1988 academic year levels. 2. Increase the capacity of schools of professional nursing. Enroll more students by (a) increasing the size of faculties and (b) increasing the number of clinical practice sites. 3. Improve the ability of the nursing educational system to respond more quickly to demand for RNs in the health care system. 4. Expand or develop new programs in specialty areas of nursing that are experiencing acute shortages, for example, nurse midwifery, public health practitioners, and nurse anesthetists. 5. Have adequate kinds and numbers of nurses available for health delivery systems in Texas. 6. Develop a manpower data system that will project the future needs of Texas's health delivery system for nurses so that the educational system can respond appropriately. 7. Assist employers of nurses to identify potential markets for recruitment. 8. Schools of nursing should ensure that at least one school of nursing per region is offering a refresher course at all times. 9. Assist employers of nurses to focus on retention of their currently employed RNs. 10. Assist employers to make better use of the registered nurses currently in employment. 11. Maximize the skills of nurse executives in institutions throughout Texas so they may effectively deal with shortage problems and demands of the health market. 12. Optimize nursing compensation and benefits to effect retention in as well as recruitment into the field of nursing. 13. The overall goal for nursing data collection activities should be to develop a nursing manpower data system for Texas that would

14. Initiate a system for collection, tabulation, and analysis of nurse manpower data that integrates nursing employment data, nursing practice data, and nursing education data.
15. Provide for compatibility of data collected by establishing a basic minimum data set for the collection of nursing manpower information in Texas.
16. Select a nursing manpower model(s) to use to project the future nursing requirements for Texas.

Vacancy rates—
Hospitals report 12.2% vacant RN staff positions and 6.6% vacant LVN positions.

RN education profile—
In 1987, 45% of new RNs were graduates of B.S.N programs; 53% were graduates of A.D.N and diploma programs.

Salaries (1988)—
Starting salary of staff RNs is $20,424 and average maximum salary is $27,960. RN salary progression is 36.9%. Starting salary of staff LVNs is $13,520 and the average maximum salary is $18,699—a salary progression of 38.3%.

Licensure data—
90% of new RN licenses were awarded to graduates of Texas programs in 1988. In 1988, in-migration of RNs into Texas was less (440 RNs and 82 LVNs) than migrated out.

Nurse/patient ratios—
Hospitals increased the proportion of RNs employed from 56% in 1981 to 65% in 1986 and the proportion of LVNs from 6.5 per 100 beds to 8.0 per 100 beds.
1,065 nursing homes with 111,516 beds: Ratio is 1.75 RN and 9.3 LVNs per 100 beds in Texas.

SOURCE: Based on data from *Texas Nursing Shortage* (1988).

53

TABLE 3.5 Nebraska: Legislative Bill 890

Purpose, Method, and Findings	Recommendations

Method:
A Nursing Education Advisory Committee was authorized to develop a preliminary plan for nursing education in the state.
 	
Findings:
Employment status—
90% nurses working full- or part-time;
53% full-time and almost half part-time
 	
Work setting (1987)—
69% FTE RNs in hospitals   5.6% FTE RNs in community health
9.6% FTE RNs in nursing homes 52% FTE LPNs in hospitals
6.5% FTE RNs in offices   26% FTE LPNs in nursing homes
 	
Increase in RN FTE (1980-1987)
18% in hospitals   30% office
48% nursing homes   50% community health
 	
Vacancy rates (1988)—
hospitals, 10% RNs, 8% LPNs; nursing homes, 15% RNs
 	
Salary—
average hourly rates in 1987: RNs, $9.73-$11.22; LPNs, $6.94-$7.91.
 	
Educational programs—
annual cost of education per FTE student
RNs, $5,151-$12,972
LPNs, $3,000-$4,765
 	
Educational graduations—
RNs, 631 in 1983, 287 in 1988
LPNs, 304 in 1987
	1. To meet the diverse educational needs of the citizens of Nebraska desiring nursing education, options should be available for
	   —all levels of educational programs
	   —with geographic accessibility
	   —with educational mobility with maximum transfer of credit
	   —with flexibility of scheduling
	   —with choice of cost
	2. Universities and colleges should ensure that their programs meet the needs of students and health care institutions of Nebraska.
	3. Financial incentives should be provided to encourage recruitment and retention of qualified individuals in programs.
	4. To make nursing a more attractive career choice, employees of nurses should be encouraged to give at least as much attention to retention of nurses as to recruitment.
	5. Focus and intensify recruitment of men and ethnic minorities into nursing. Public media should assist in providing an accurate image of the challenges and opportunities of nursing.
	6. The Nebraska Assembly of Nursing Deans and Directors should be encouraged and supported by state funds to coordinate planning for maximum educational mobility for nurses.
	7. Availability and access to graduate education in nursing are mandatory to provide adequately prepared faculty, nursing service administrators, and a supply of clinical specialists.

8. New programs should not be authorized without adequate documentation of geographic need, adequate facilities, and impact on existing programs.
9. The state should consider contracting for slots within existing programs as an alternative to funding new programs.
10. Technical community colleges should be the primary public delivery agent for the associate degree in nursing.
11. Nursing education and practice in Nebraska should continue to be of high quality and should not be compromised because of the nursing shortage.

SOURCE: *Nebraska Nurse Education Plan* (1989).

TABLE 3.6 North Carolina: Authorized by Chapter 1049 (HB 2461) of the 1987 Session Laws

Purpose, Method, and Findings	*Recommendations (partial listing)*

Purpose:
To study the issues regarding the nursing shortage and to propose long-term solutions to the General Assembly
Method:
  Created Legislative Study Commission on Nursing
Findings:
  Supply—
    54,000 RNs licensed
    19,000 LPNs licensed
  Work setting—
    66% of RNs work in hospitals
  Employment status—
    80% of RNs employed in nursing
    76% of LPNs employed in nursing
  Educational enrollments and graduations—
    Enrollment declined 22% in RN programs and 45% in LPN programs between 1983 and 1987.
  Licensure data—
    Numbers taking exam decreased 27% from 1984 to 1988. Failure rates increased 31% from 1984 to 1988.
	1. The Department of Community Colleges and the baccalaureate schools of nursing should be encouraged to improve the transferability of credits taken for the A.D.N. to the baccalaureate program.
	2. The Department of Community Colleges should expand offering A.D.N. programs at employment sites for LPNs.
	3. Baccalaureate schools of nursing should examine efforts to provide on-campus B.S.N. programs for working RNs.
	4. The commission recommends a multilevel scholarship program to attract bright people and nontraditional students and adults into nursing and to provide increased financial aid for nursing students.
	5. High school guidance counselors should receive health occupation marketing materials and information.
	6. Per student funding for nursing programs in community colleges should be increased.
	7. Increase salaries of community college and UNC nursing instructors to compete for and attract additional instructors to meet program needs.
	8. A comprehensive, generic professional media campaign on nursing as a profession should be developed and funded over two years.

9. Schools of nursing in community colleges and the UNC shall review curriculum structure and schedules to ensure flexibility and access for nontraditional students.

10. Retention of nurses should be increased by providing state funding to employers for innovations in retaining direct care nurses, offering greater flexibility and choice in fringe benefits, and integrating clinical ladders with educational advancement and salary levels.

11. The General Assembly should provide funds for planning for a Center for Excellence in Nursing.

12. The range in base pay must be expanded from the 25%-30% now prevalent to at least 75%-85%.

13. The counties must be encouraged to keep pay for public health nurses competitive with salary levels for other nurse employers.

14. Employers and nurses must explore ways to increase productivity of nursing time.

SOURCE: *Final Report: The Legislature Study Commission on Nursing* (1989).

TABLE 3.7 Tennessee

Purpose, Method, and Findings	Recommendations (partial listing)
Purpose: (a) Evaluate nursing in the current health care environment (b) Bring recommendations concerning any needed change in the legal statutes governing nursing, the educational preparation of nurses, and the programs needed to provide an adequately prepared supply of nurses to meet the consumer needs of Tennessee Method: Statewide master planning commission on nursing practice and education; public meetings for written and oral testimony Findings: Supply— 25,300 RNs in 1984 19,772 LPNs in 1983 Work setting— hospitals 79.4% RNs 8.7% LPNs 12.0% aides nursing homes 16% RNs 22.9% LPNs 61% aides community health 34.3% RNs 65.7% aides Employment status— 88.5% RNs employed in nursing Educational profile— In 1984, 25,300 RNs in Tennessee 17,320 A.D.N./diploma 5,980 B.S.N. 2,010 graduate level	1. Tennessee Nurses' Association should foster and assist in public relations and marketing efforts to enhance the nursing image and to encourage existing and potential students into the career. 2. The role of the nursing professional should be strengthened within health care facilities whereby there would be more decision making in terms of patient care policies. 3. Support should be given to alternative delivery systems managed and/or staffed by nurses. 4. Compensation should be commensurate with responsibility, prior professional experience, level of clinical competence, and length of service. 5. Mechanisms to facilitate transition from education to workplace such as effective orientation programs and internships should be encouraged. 6. Demonstration projects should be designed that address work environment factors that influence recruitment and retention. 7. A formal network should be established by health care-related organizations for nursing service administrators, clinicians, educators, and researchers to cooperate in conducting multisite nursing research and in sharing findings. 8. A multidisciplinary research center for health sciences should be established at a state university and be supported chiefly from funds that are now used to engage private consultants and private researchers for state projects. 9. Funding support should be given to demonstration of innovations in nursing practice, education, and administration, especially new areas where professional nurse activities may improve health outcomes and/or affect cost containment. 10. The current supply of graduates of nursing programs should be maintained but emphasis should be given to increasing the

Employment projections (2000)—
45,510 FTE RNs
8,355 FTE LPNs
32,574 FTE aides
Need for FTE RNs
63.3% for hospitals
8.0% for community health
8.8% for physicians ambulatory care
3.0% for schools of nursing
0.4% for health-related organizations
Need for FTE LPNs
37.8% for hospitals
62.2% for nursing home
Need for FTE aides
13.3% for hospitals
42.6% for nursing homes
44.1% for community health
Educational projections—
1.5% of RNs should be prepared at the doctoral level
20.2% should be prepared at the master's level
48.4% should be prepared at the B.S.N. level
29.9% should be prepared at the A.D.N./diploma level
32.6% of master's prepared nurses should have nurse practitioner preparation

geographic and financial accessibility to nursing programs of baccalaureate and higher degrees across the state.

11. In terms of funding, where possible, existing programs should be expanded.

12. Community colleges should be encouraged to develop prenursing programs that articulate with baccalaureate programs.

13. The number of baccalaureate programs should be increased by 50% and total enrollments in baccalaureate programs be at least doubled over current enrollment.

14. The current number of associate degree programs should be maintained and total enrollments increased 15% over current enrollment.

15. The number of practical nursing programs should be decreased by 3% and total enrollments should be decreased by 40% below current enrollments.

16. An organized statewide effort should be implemented and directed at recruitment of students into the nursing profession.

17. Scholarships and financial aid must be available where applicable and payback mechanisms should be used with the requirements that the recipients work in underserved areas for specified periods of time.

18. Nursing education should be more accessible to qualified "nontraditional" students and to nurses who wish to advance their education.

19. Financial support should be made available to support school efforts to design and implement innovative nursing programs to meet the needs of minorities, gifted, and disadvantaged students.

20. Mechanisms should be developed by the year 2000 to track nursing's contribution to health care cost containment and revenue generation and to provide third party reimbursement for nursing services.

SOURCE: *Tennessee Plan for Nursing for the Year 2000* (1987).

59

TABLE 3.8 Pennsylvania: House Resolution No. 195

Purpose, Method, and Findings	Recommendations (partial listing)
Purpose of study: (a) Develop plan of action to describe the problems created by the shortage (b) Make recommendations regarding recruitment and creation of environment that would increase retention of nurses Method: A legislative task force was formed, and two hearings were conducted. Findings: Vacancy rates (1986)— 3.8% long term care 6.8% acute care 3.5% home health care Vacancy rates (last 6 months of 1987)— 4.4% long term care 8.1% acute care 4.3% home health care Salary— average maximum RN salary is $29,000 Education programs— 31 B.S.N. programs 22 A.D.N. programs 35 diploma programs 50 LPN programs Licensure data— 1987—2,112 new RNs 1987—5,090 RNs endorsed out	1. Make changes in state government to enhance the supply of nurses, including conducting a biannual survey of RNs and LPNs, establishing a Director of Public Health Nursing, and studying whether all health care personnel licensing boards should be combined into one board. 2. Propose regulations to allow LPNs to engage in additional scope of practice that is consistent with their training. 3. Expand pool of nurses by helping part-time nurses return to full-time, using educational outreach programs, facilitating educational mobility, increasing financial aid to career changers, and giving six-month work permits to new graduates of accredited state schools. 4. Remove reimbursement barriers to health employers to foster competitive salaries and benefits for nurses. 5. Improve recruitment and retention of nurses by providing salaries based on educational investment, establishing career ladders, offering on-site day care, removing housekeeping functions from nursing responsibilities, and providing opportunities for nurses to serve on committees and boards. 6. Provide financial assistance in form of scholarship and loan forgiveness programs for nursing students and increase work study programs and educational flexibility. 7. Upgrade faculty expertise in care of elderly and other long-term care patients. 8. Enhance the recruitment of nurses by developing public media campaigns promoting nursing career choice and nursing image, establishing a Governors School for Health Care Careers, and organizing computerized job data bank on a regional basis.

SOURCE: *Report of the Task Force on the Nursing Shortage* (1988).

FOUR

Supply and Demand Trends

WILLIAM J. SEROW

There has recently emerged a considerable body of literature dealing with the perceived shortage in the supply of professional nurses in the United States, which not only reflects a concern for the current situation but, perhaps even more important, views future prospects with a considerable degree of alarm. Recent extensive reviews of the professional literature on this subject (Carlson & Cowart, 1988; Speake, 1988), while expressing considerable concern over the appropriate means to measure current shortages, reveal numerous factors that have changed in the recent past and that are likely to continue to change into the foreseeable future. Such changes will influence both the demand for and the supply of professional nursing personnel.

Changes on the demand side may be linked to changes in the demographic structure of the entire population (particularly with regard to age and race/ethnicity); changes in the characteristics of the patient population (including not only the well-documented increase in the number of old and very old persons [Serow & Sly, 1988] but also, among other things, increases in such phenomena as persons with histories of substance abuse and the emergence of AIDS as a critical public health problem); changes in the delivery of health care (including marked advances in biomedical technology and changes in institutional arrangements regarding patterns of patient care and more intensive use of professional nurses in a broad array of functions); and changes in health care finance policies, which are simultaneously reducing the average length of stay and increasing the degree of morbidity among the hospitalized population. At least in the short run, it is likely that the interplay of these factors will increase the demand for professional nurses. For our purposes here, it is important to understand that many of these factors will serve to establish national

61

parameters but will have little if any effect on the distribution of demand for nurses across states. This is generally the case for health care delivery and financing issues. Furthermore, it is likely that projections of demographic parameters, such as age, gender, and race or ethnicity, will capture not only differential demand across states for nursing services that might be viewed as being highly specific to some segment of the population (obstetrics and long-term care, for example) but also differential demand arising from conditions such as AIDS or those seen as growing out of substance abuse.

On the supply side, Carlson and Cowart (1988) and Speake (1988) have identified two primary factors that have acted and are likely to continue to act at least to reduce the rate of increase in the number of professional nurses. The first is really a complex set of factors pertaining to job satisfaction/dissatisfaction including salary/benefit issues, working conditions, and perceived professionalization. The second is decreased enrollment in nursing education programs, which may, in turn, be related to both demographic (reduced numbers of college-age persons) and economic (relatively low earnings in nursing compared with other health and non-health-related alternatives) considerations.

Certainly, the evidence amassed by Carlson and Cowart and by Speake supports the hypothesis that the national imbalance between demand and supply in the nursing profession is mirrored in Florida. They report that a study conducted by the Florida Health Care Association and the Florida Association of Homes for the Aged found nursing vacancy rates of 7% to 17% in 1987 (depending upon institutional setting), while a study conducted in the same year by the Florida Hospital Association found an overall vacancy rate of 10.4% for registered nurse positions in contrast to an 11.1% rate found in a previous (1982) study by the same organization and a 13.6% rate reported nationally the previous December (Curran, Minnick, & Moss, 1987). The work of the Florida Hospital Association also showed appreciably lower vacancy rates for LPN and nurse aide positions (6.1% and 5.5%, respectively) than for RNs.

By objective criteria, the supply of professional nurses in Florida has been expanding in recent years. For example, the total number of active licenses for registered nurses in the state rose from 55,747 in 1975 to 96,185 as of May 12, 1987 (American Nurses Association, various years; Florida Department of Health and Rehabilitative Services, 1988). The observed increase of 63.8% in Florida between 1975 and 1985 far exceeded the 24.0% recorded at the national level.

Additionally, data from the American Hospital Association (1983-1987) show that the full-time equivalent number of registered nurses employed in Florida's hospitals rose by 15.6% during the four-year period beginning in 1982 (from 34,401 to 39,758).

Data on the employment of licensed practical nurses in Florida are somewhat more limited in scope. The number of active licenses rose from 31,299 in 1980 to 33,403 in 1987 (Bureau of Economic and Business Research, 1980, 1987), but the number employed in this capacity fell from 21,721 in 1985 to 20,263 in 1987 (Florida State Board of Nursing, 1988). If we consider only the number of LPNs employed in hospitals, their number rose from 9,136 in 1976 to a peak of 12,711 in 1982 before declining to 9,184 in 1986 (American Hospital Association, 1977-1987).

As an indicator of prospective future growth in the supply of nurses in the state, one need first and foremost consider recent trends in the production of registered and practical nurses, that is, data pertaining to graduation from and enrollment in training programs that prepare one for a career as a nurse. Here, the trends are somewhat less sanguine. Data from the Florida State Board of Nursing (1988) suggest that the number of graduations from programs training individuals to become registered nurses rose from a level of 2,600-2,700 at the beginning of the 1980s to some 3,200 at mid-decade but have fallen by some 15% to 20% thereafter, so that there is little difference between initial and current levels. A similar pattern may be observed with reference to the pattern of graduates from practical nurse programs, with the exception that the decline during the past few years has been nearly 50%, so that current levels are less than two thirds of what they were at the beginning of the decade.

The remainder of this chapter will be devoted to a review of the methodology and results of a recently published national-level assessment of the future course of supply and demand for professional nursing personnel (U.S. Department of Health and Human Services [DHHS], 1988) in Florida and the United States as a whole, followed by presentation and discussion of an alternative approach to the allocation of projected national totals to the state level.

Projection Methodology

The tenth chapter of the *Sixth Report to the President and Congress on the Status of Health Personnel* is devoted to the nursing profession.

In essence, this document represents the "state of the art" in terms of appropriate methodologies for the projection of the supply of and demand for nurses in the United States as a whole and in each individual state. As is true for all projection exercises, the results are very sensitive to the assumptions made on the course of future events that are thought to have an impact on the variables being forecast. Additionally, it may be stated as a rule of thumb that forecasts for small areas are prone to relatively greater error than are forecasts for larger areas and that forecasts for more remote points in time are prone to relatively greater error than are forecasts for more proximate points in time (Irwin, 1977).

In general, models developed to forecast the *supply* of nurses in the United States are designed to capture the dynamics of the flow of nurses into and out of licensure and the work force. Trend data on labor market behavior are developed from recurrent surveys of nurses (the 1977, 1980, and 1984 National Sample Surveys of Registered Nurses and the 1983 National Sample Survey of Licensed Practical/Vocational Nurses) as well as from current projections of the national and state populations (specific to age and gender) prepared on a regular basis by the U.S. Bureau of the Census (e.g., Wetrogan, 1988). In the case of LPNs, sampling variability is so great in smaller states that no state-level projections were prepared. For the case of registered nurses, two alternative projections ("Series A" and "Series B") have been prepared. These differ largely with respect to the supply of nurses trained by baccalaureate programs. Series A represents current concerns about decreasing enrollments in these programs and, accordingly, represents a "constrained" picture based on survey data compiled by the American Association of Colleges of Nursing (1987). By way of contrast, Series B is simply a continuation of enrollment and labor market trends observed during the past few years.

A total of four alternative projections of the demand for nursing personnel are included in the DHHS report. There are two alternative approaches (the so-called Historical Trend-Based Model and the Criteria-Based Model), each of which includes two variants.

The Historical Trend-Based Model produces projections based on trends in three major variables: demographics (particularly age and gender) of the population; provided services (such as inpatient days, outpatient visits, and the like) per capita; and the number of full-time equivalent RNs and LPNs per unit of provided service. In the so-called *baseline* variant of the historical trends model, the dominant assumption is that these trends will continue throughout the planning horizon, subject to some judgmental modification as a result of changes in the system of health care delivery consequent to cost containment strategies initiated both within the industry and in response to changes in federal government reimbursement policy. The other variant within this overall approach is termed the *case management* approach; this results from the decreasing rate of hospital admissions as health care needs that would previously have led to an admission now may be treated in other health care settings. Such an approach is very consistent with the observed expansion of home health care, low-intensity nursing care facilities, health maintenance organizations, and outpatient surgery.

The alternative Criteria-Based Model may be viewed as being somewhat more complex, in that nursing requirements are determined by the number of nursing personnel, divided by level of educational attainment, necessary to meet a particular set of health care goals. These criteria were established and are updated by a panel of experts, based upon reviews of past and current practices and experiences. The most recent revision of the criteria was accomplished in 1987 (see Kearns, 1987), and it is these revisions that underlie the projections reproduced below. These criteria-based projections are also prepared with two variants, termed the *lower* and the *upper bound*. The lower bound is assumed to be the level all states would achieve, while the upper bound is the level that some states *could* achieve and toward which all other states *would* work. Criteria, both lower bound and upper bound, are formulated for the years 2000, 2010, and 2020 and are quite specific with regard to numbers and types of nurses required to deliver specified types of services.

Existing Projections of Demand for Florida and the United States

Figure 4.1 shows what could be termed the *baseline* data, that is, the (full-time equivalent) number of registered nurses and licensed practical nurses in both Florida and the United States. For RNs, the data are from 1984; for LPNs, 1983 data were the most current at the time of the preparation of the BHP report. These data show that Florida had a marginally larger share of the nation's RNs (4.71%) in

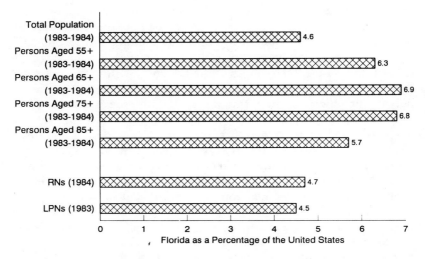

Figure 4.1. The Relative Size of Population and Professional Nurses in Florida and the United States (1983 and 1984)

1984 than it did of the nation's population in the same year (4.67%; U.S. Bureau of the Census, 1989); for LPNs, in the preceding year, there was again approximate equality between the state's share of nurses and its share of total population, but, in this instance, the latter was marginally greater than the former (4.59% and 4.47%, respectively). It is useful to consider the observed time trend of these ratios. In 1977, for example, Florida accounted for 4.03% of both the nation's population and its registered nurses. In 1973, Florida accounted for some 3.21% of the nation's LPNs and 3.74% of its total population (Byerly, 1984; U.S. DHHS, 1982). In other words, one can observe that, in the recent past, Florida's number of nurses of both types has grown relative to that of the United States at a rate exceeding that of total population (relative to the nation as a whole).

One should also note from the 1983-1984 data that the state's share of national nursing personnel, while equal to that of total population, is much less than its share of the older population, however defined. While Florida accounted for about 5% of all nurses in the United States, it accounted for some 6%-7% of the nation's older citizens. Census data from 1970 and 1980 show that Florida accounted for 3.3% and 4.3% (respectively) of total population but for 5.0% and 6.6% of those

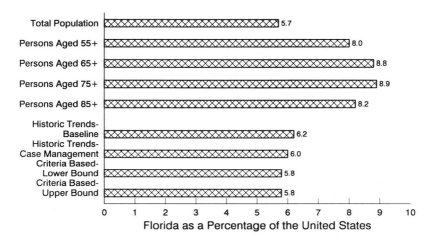

Figure 4.2. The Relative Size of Population and the Demand for Registered Nurses (Florida and the United States—2000)

aged 65 and over. These shares stood at 4.7% and 6.9% in 1984. If one were to assume that the observed increase in Florida's share of the nation's elderly during the 1970s occurred at a constant rate, its share of those aged 65 and over in 1977 would have stood at 6.0%. Thus, between 1977 and 1984, Florida's actual *share* of the nation's registered nurses increased at an average annual rate of 2.25% per year, slightly exceeding that of the state's share of total national population (2.13%) or of the elderly (2.08%).

Figures 4.2 and 4.3 present data pertaining to the demand for nurses in Florida and in the United States for the year 2000. During the period from the mid-1980s until the turn of the century, population projections suggest that Florida's share of the national population would rise from 4.6% to 5.7%, while its share of registered nurses would increase from the initial level of 4.7% to a range of 5.8% (both variants of the criteria-based model) to 6.2% (historic trends-baseline). The state's share of LPNs, however, actually is projected to decline during the period. Finally, projections of the state's share of the nation's older population suggest an increase from the 6%-7% level to one of 8%-9%. In sum, during the period from 1983-1984 until the year 2000, the projections show the relative

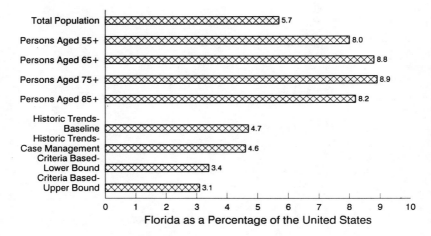

Figure 4.3. The Relative Size of Population and the Demand for Licensed Practical Nurses (Florida and the United States—2000)

demand for registered nurses rising at a rate exceeding that of the total population in all projection variants but lagging behind the growth rate for the share of the older population. In all cases, Florida's share of LPNs is forecast to decline.

Figure 4.4 and 4.5 present data pertaining to the demand for nurses in Florida and in the United States for the year 2020. During the period from the turn of the century until 2020, population projections suggest that Florida's share of the national population would rise from 5.7% to 6.5%, while its share of registered nurses would increase from the initial level of about 6.0% to a range of 5.7% (historic trends-case management) to 6.5% (historic trends-baseline). Thus, in all but one case, the state's share of total population is forecast to exceed that for registered nurses. Furthermore, the state's share of LPNs is projected to decline still more during the period to levels of 3.7% to 3.9% (only the historic trends model is used in this instance). Finally, projections of the state's share of the nation's older population suggest an increase from the 8%-9% level to one of 9%-10%, with appreciably higher levels to be observed among the very old. In sum, during the period from 2000 until the year 2020, the projections show the relative demand for registered nurses rising at a rate less than or (in only one case) equal to that of

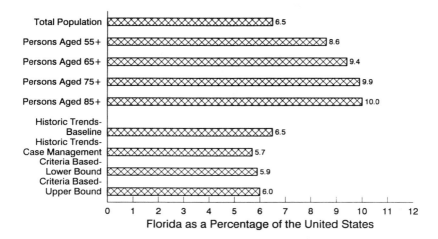

Figure 4.4. The Relative Size of Population and the Demand for Registered Nurses (Florida and the United States—2020)

total population in all projection variants but still lagging behind the growth rate for the share of the older population. In all cases, Florida's share of LPNs is forecast to continue to decline.

From these results, I suggest that the perceived difficulties with the BHP projections are most pronounced for the case of LPNs and, to a lesser extent, for RNs after the year 2000. In reviewing the data sources identified in the BHP projections, it is unclear whether population trends below the national level after 1985 were considered in the projection process. More specifically, the data used are identified as national-level projections (using the most recent then available) and current state-level population estimates to the year 1985. It is unclear whether states were implicitly assumed to maintain their 1985 share or somehow to continue to increase relative growth/decline at some preexisting level, but, in any case, there does not appear to have been any effort to consider growth differentials among states, especially with regard to changes in age structure.

Putting the matter in a slightly different context, I suggest that the problem with the BHP projections may not be a question of methodology or results at the national level but a question of the absence of a clearly defined and tested methodology of allocation of

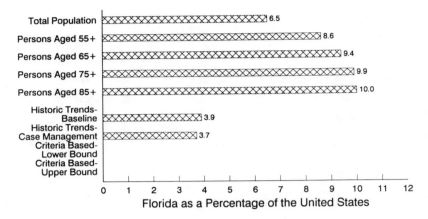

Figure 4.5. The Relative Size of Population and the Demand for Licensed Practical Nurses (Florida and the United States—2020)
NOTE: Criteria-based projections were not prepared for licensed practical nurses.

national-level projections to the state level. In this regard, the changing demography of Florida vis-à-vis the remainder of the nation is quite germane. Table 4.1 presents data on the estimated (1984) and projected population of both Florida and the United States, by age and gender, for the years 2000 and 2020. These data show that Florida's share of the total U.S. population is forecast to rise from the estimated level of 4.7% in 1984 to some 6.5% by the end of the projection period. During the entire 36-year period, Florida's population is projected to increase by nearly 73%, from an initial level of 11.1 million to 19.1 million. For the entire country, the rate of population increase is a comparatively low 24%, from 236.5 to 292.6 million. Thus, of the total national population increase of 56.1 million persons, some 8.1 million (or 14%) is forecast to occur within Florida.

As is well known, Florida is the oldest state of all 50, in terms of share of population aged 65 or over or in terms of median age of the population. In 1984, for example, some 17.5% of Florida's population was at least 65 years old in contrast to 11.8% for the entire country. In 1984, the median age of Florida's population was 35.6 years in contrast to the level of 31.1 years for the entire United States. By the end of the projection period in 2020, more than one fourth of Florida's population and more than one sixth of the nation's pop-

TABLE 4.1 Population Estimates and Projections for the United States and Florida: 1984, 2000, and 2020 (thousands of persons)

Year	Age	United States		Florida		Florida as a Percentage of United States	
		Female	Total	Female	Total	Female	Total
1984	0-4	8,708	17,830	349	714	4.01	4.00
	5-14	16,580	33,975	650	1,332	3.92	3.92
	15-24	19,873	40,113	832	1,672	4.19	4.17
	25-34	20,663	41,231	862	1,712	4.17	4.15
	35-44	15,526	30,546	683	1,330	4.40	4.35
	45-54	11,581	22,494	563	1,078	4.86	4.79
	55-64	11,841	22,316	701	1,275	5.92	5.71
	65-74	9,409	16,740	646	1,171	6.87	7.00
	75-84	5,411	8,616	360	616	6.65	7.15
	85+	1,863	2,615	99	152	5.31	5.81
	Total	121,455	236,476	5,745	11,052	4.73	4.67
2000	0-4	8,237	16,898	398	813	4.83	4.81
	5-14	18,194	37,334	903	1,847	4.96	4.95
	15-24	18,028	36,468	893	1,794	4.95	4.92
	25-34	18,465	36,952	933	1,844	5.05	4.99
	35-44	21,964	43,841	1,169	2,297	5.32	5.24
	45-54	18,927	37,216	1,085	2,091	5.73	5.62
	55-64	12,601	24,158	888	1,662	7.05	6.88
	65-74	10,001	18,243	855	1,590	8.55	8.72
	75-84	7,307	12,017	627	1,098	8.58	9.14
	85+	3,300	4,622	253	381	7.67	8.24
	Total	137,024	267,749	8,004	15,417	5.84	5.76
2020	0-4	8,181	16,794	421	859	5.14	5.11
	5-14	16,798	34,507	887	1,815	5.28	5.26
	15-24	17,412	35,278	955	1,919	5.49	5.44
	25-34	19,477	39,040	1,074	2,123	5.52	5.44
	35-44	18,843	37,601	1,076	2,115	5.71	5.62
	45-54	18,453	36,587	1,190	2,293	6.45	6.27
	55-64	20,979	41,064	1,656	3,099	7.89	7.55
	65-74	16,428	30,805	1,517	2,821	9.23	9.16
	75-84	8,379	14,205	812	1,422	9.69	10.01
	85+	4,745	6,730	441	664	9.29	9.87
	Total	149,695	292,611	10,029	19,130	6.70	6.54

SOURCE: U.S. Bureau of the Census (1989), Wetrogan (1988), and the author's calculations.

ulation will be at least 64 years of age (25.7% and 17.7%, respectively). The median age will have risen to 48.3 years in Florida and to 40.3 years for the United States as a whole. During this period, Florida's share of the nation's older population (aged 65+) will have risen from 6.9% to 9.4% and its share of the very old population (aged 85+) from 5.8% to 10.0%. Collectively, the nation's elderly will grow in numbers from 28.0 to 51.7 million, or by 85%. In Florida, the number of elderly is projected to rise from 1.9 to 4.9 million, or by 153%. Finally, the number of very old persons in the United States will rise by 157% (from 2.6 to 6.7 million) and in Florida by 337% (from 152,000 to 664,000).

In light of these comparative demographic trends, it seems reasonable to assert that the demand-side projections for nurses in Florida may understate the actual magnitude of requirements. I have argued that there may be difficulties with the initial data used, specifically in terms of the projections' allocation of nursing demand to individual states. This chapter will now describe a model that might serve to better allocate the national numbers and report on the results stemming from an initial estimation of this model.

An Alternative Model for the Allocation of Nursing Demand

The model I propose for use here is one that stems from the demographic literature, particularly that pertaining to population estimation and projection. The particular model is termed *difference correlation* and is used to allocate the value of the variable in question to the (exhaustive) components of some predetermined total (O'Hare, 1976). A variant of this model (*ratio correlation*) is used by the U.S. Bureau of the Census to allocate state-level populations from predetermined national totals and by state agencies to allocate county-level populations from predetermined state totals. The basic paradigm of the model is that changes in each component's share of the dependent variable are functionally related to changes in the component's share of the so-called coincident indicators. In estimating total population, for example, one could hypothesize that changes in variables such as the share of births, deaths, tax returns, automobile registrations, school enrollments, voter registrations, and the like would explain much of the variation in changes in the respective shares of population. In the model to be described and tested here, I hypothesize that changes in each state's share of the projected demand for nurses will be functionally related to changes in each state's share of population variables. I will report here only on the simpler case, where I estimate a single variable model, relating changes in the share of demand for nurses to changes in the share of total population. An alternative (multivariate) specification was also developed (incorporating age, gender, and racial components of the population) but it failed to provide a better fitting and therefore more reliable model.

The model is first estimated for observed changes over time: In the case of registered nurses, the dependent variable is the change in each state's share of registered nurses between 1977 and 1984, while the independent, or explanatory, variables are changes in population shares for the same time period. In the case of LPNs, the time horizon is 1973 to 1983. For the model to work in the forecast mode, it is necessary to assume that the estimated coefficients remain stable over time. Clearly, this is a critical assumption of this model but perhaps one that is least amenable to empirical verification. Such an assumption is, of course, commonplace in many forecasting approaches, including several developed specifically for the nursing labor market (see Deane & Ro, 1979). In any event, once the coefficients of the model are determined, the projected values of the independent variables for each state (in the years 2000 and 2020) are substituted into the equation, and the equation is then "solved" for each state. The outcome is each state's projected share of the appropriate total (i.e., projected national demand for registered nurses or LPNs). After these are adjusted to account for the differing time horizon between the estimated and forecast periods, and controls are imposed to ensure that the forecast sum of state-level shares equals 100%, the final result (state-level projections of demand) is obtained simply by multiplying the forecast share for each state by the appropriate projected national total.

The estimated equation for registered nurses is

$$\text{RNDIF} = -.0000003 + 1.083 \text{ RPOPDIF} \qquad [1]$$

$$(t = 6.3) \; R^2 = .444; \; F = 39.1$$

and that for LPNs is

$$\text{LPNDIF} = -.0000002 + 0.793 \text{ LPOPDIF} \qquad [2]$$

$$(t = 4.2) \ R^2 = .264; \ F = 17.6$$

where RNDIF is the difference for each state in its share of the nation's RNs between 1977 and 1984; RPOPDIF is the difference for each state in its share of the nation's population between 1977 and 1984; LPNDIF is the difference for each state in its share of the nation's LPNs between 1974 and 1983; and LPOPDIF is the difference for each state in its share of the nation's population between 1974 and 1983.

Each equation is statistically significant in terms of its overall level of explanatory power (the value of R^2) and the value of the coefficient of the population variable. Each equation is then solved for the years 2000 and 2020 by inserting the values of the known differences in shares of the national population between 1983 (1984) and 2000 and between 2000 and 2020:

$$RNRAT00 = RN \ 84 - .0000003 + 1.083 \ (POP00\text{-}POP84) \qquad [3]$$

$$LPNRAT00 = LPN \ 83 - .0000002 + 0.793 \ (POP00\text{-}POP83) \qquad [4]$$

$$RNRAT20 = RNRAT00 - .0000003 + 1.083 \ (POP20\text{-}POP00) \qquad [5]$$

$$LPNRAT20 = LPNRAT00 - .0000002 + 0.793 \ (POP20\text{-}POP00) \qquad [6]$$

where RNRAT00(20) is each state's predicted share of the nation's demand for registered nurses in 2000 (2020); LPNRAT00(20) is each state's predicted share of the nation's demand for LPNs in 2000 (2020); RN 84 is each state's actual share of the nation's demand for registered nurses in 1984; LPN 83 is each state's actual share of the nation's demand for LPNs in 1983; POP83(84)(00)(20) is each state's actual or projected share of the nation's population in 1983, 1984, 2000, or 2020.

The results of the application of these models to the national-level forecasts of BHP yield an alternative scheme of allocation of the national totals. Table 4.2 presents the results for Florida.

These alternative projections seem, in general, to be more consistent with projected changes in Florida's share of the national population, while, at the same time, not really representing a radical departure from the BHP forecasts (especially in the case of RNs). For the year 2000, the RN projections shown here are within 5% of those made by BHP and, in the case of the historic trend variants, are below those of BHP. In this year, this projection shows Florida's

TABLE 4.2 Alternative Projections of the Demand for Professional
Nurses in Florida: 2000 and 2020

Year	BHP		Alternative		Percentage Difference	
	LPNs	RNs	LPNs	RNs	LPNs	RNs
2000						
Historic trends:						
baseline	27,460	108,250	31,585	102,504	15.0	−5.3
Historic trends:						
case management	26,090	99,500	30,765	97,065	17.9	−2.4
Criteria based:						
lower bound	9,970	104,590	15,737	106,846	57.8	2.2
Criteria based:						
upper bound	8,910	132,420	15,639	133,441	75.5	0.8
2020						
Historic trends:						
baseline	35,700	155,020	55,155	160,660	54.5	3.6
Historic trends:						
case management	30,960	105,680	50,261	124,488	62.3	17.8
Criteria based:						
lower bound	—	203,440	—	229,569	—	12.8
Criteria based:						
upper bound	—	247,700	—	274,770	—	10.9

share of RNs at 5.9% of the national level, up from 4.7% in 1984; the state's share of LPNs rises from 4.5% in 1983 to 5.4%. During this period, Florida's share of total population rose from 4.6% or 4.7% to 5.8%. In 2020, this forecast of the share of RNs and LPNs suggests an increase to 6.7% and 6.0%, respectively. The share of population is projected to be 6.5%.

The foregoing remarks should not be taken as an unequivocal assertion that one version of the model will prove more accurate than the other or, for that matter, that the approach to forecasting demand for professional nurses that is introduced here will necessarily prove to be more accurate than that of BHP or any other approach. The proof of the reliability of a forecast can only be developed at the end of the forecast period. The approach taken here certainly yields results that are more consistent with projected levels of population change at the state level, but one must realize that the caveats made regarding the comparative accuracy of forecasts of demand apply equally to forecasts of demographic variables. The latter, however, necessarily underlie the former. The results presented here are more consistent with the underlying demographic trends than are those of the BHP.

Conclusion

One might argue that the approach taken here is too mechanical in that it ignores the dynamics that are occurring within the health care industry. I assert that these dynamics are in fact embodied in the national-level forecasts developed by BHP and that the critical issue from our perspective is the means of allocation of the national control figures to the state level. Whether the dynamics are in fact properly accounted for at the national level is also a question that can only be resolved over the course of time. One would hope that changes in the use of professional nurses and in the roles they play in health care, especially in hospitals and nursing homes, will become embodied in recurring rounds of projections prepared by BHP and other recognized bodies within the profession.

FIVE

The Education of Nurses

DIANNE L. SPEAKE

Overview

Enrollments in nursing education programs in this country sharply declined during the 1980s while the demand for nurses continued to rise. The National League for Nursing (1988) indicates that the number of nursing students seeking to be licensed peaked in 1983 at 250,553 but dropped 13% to 218,000 in 1985, reflecting decreases of 12% in baccalaureate (B.S.N.) programs and 19% in associate degree (A.D.N.) programs. The Secretary's Commission on Nursing predicts the gap between supply and demand will continue to widen as greater numbers of nurses leave the profession than are replaced by new graduates (U.S. Department of Health and Human Services [DHHS], 1988).

Recent data indicate that fewer students are choosing nursing as a career. Each year, the Cooperative Institutional Research Program (CIRP) at the University of California, Los Angeles, polls 300,000 full-time freshmen at 550 two- and four-year colleges and universities (Astin, 1988). In 1987, this survey indicated that only 4.0% of women freshman planned to become registered nurses—less than half the 1974 peak of 10.2%. By comparison, freshmen women are considering business (23%), teaching (11%), law (4.0%), medicine (3.4%), and engineering (2.8%). Men reported even less (0.2%) attraction to nursing. By 1991, U.S. colleges will award some 14,500 baccalaureate degrees in nursing compared with 16,000 physician or MD degrees (Mershon, 1988).

In addition, the characteristics of students choosing nursing as a career have changed. Williams's study (1988) examined data from the annual American Freshman Survey from 1966 to 1982. Williams reports declining interest in nursing among high-achieving high school students and those students from middle to upper socioeconomic groups. While interest in nursing as a career has diminished among Caucasian students, interest has increased among black students. It appears that the altruism and social concerns traditionally associated with nursing are losing ground to current student values emphasizing money, power, and status. Williams (1988) warns that, unless rewards are built into nursing education and practice, high-achieving well-prepared college students are unlikely to choose nursing as a career. In addition, the decreasing size of the 18- to 24-year-old population suggests a need to recruit nontraditional students into the profession.

The purpose of this study was to examine the variables that affect enrollments in nursing education programs in Florida. The study examined enrollment and graduation statistics, financial aid, recruitment and retention strategies, articulation and career ladder opportunities, and availability of qualified faculty.

A Nursing Education Questionnaire was developed to address these variables and was distributed in April 1989 to all LPN, RN, and graduate nursing education programs in the state. Repeat mailings were made to nonrespondents in May 1989. Responses to the questionnaire were received from 24 practical nurse (LPN) programs (71%), 18 associate degree (A.D.N.) programs (69%), 11 baccalaureate degree (B.S.N.) programs (85%), and 6 graduate programs (100%). Florida programs offering certificates for nurse anesthetists (N = 1) and nurse practitioners (N = 3) were not surveyed in this study.

TRENDS IN ENROLLMENTS AND GRADUATIONS

Enrollments in nursing programs in Florida declined 34% between 1983 and 1987. Graduations declined 17% during this time. More recent enrollment statistics indicate enrollments increased in associate degree and diploma programs in 1987-1989 but remain far below 1983-1984 enrollments (Figure 5.1). Enrollments in B.S.N. programs, however, do not reflect this reversal in the downward spiral. Enrollments in LPN programs also show gains for 1988-1989. Graduation statistics show improvements in associate degree and LPN programs but continuing declines in baccalaureate and diploma programs (Figure 5.2).

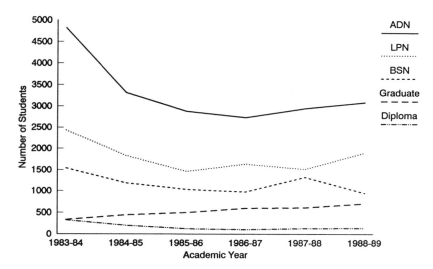

Figure 5.1. Student Enrollment in Florida Nursing Programs: Academic
Years 1983-1984 to 1988-1989
SOURCE: Florida Board of Nursing.

FINANCIAL SUPPORT AND STUDENT ASSISTANCE

Nursing education in Florida's community colleges and public
universities is financed by public funds—primarily general revenue
funds. In general, a formula reflecting the number of credit hours
awarded by each program determines the amount of general revenue funding received by each institution. The funds themselves go
to the institution as unrestricted funds, not to the nursing program
itself. The institution's administration determines the amount of
funds that the nursing program will actually receive. This amount
may be more or less than the amount the institution receives from
the general revenue funds appropriated on the basis of the formula.

LPN education in Florida occurs in community colleges (10 programs), postsecondary adult vocational centers (22 programs), private schools, and hospitals (2 programs). It is financed primarily by
public general revenue funds, by federal vocational education
grants, and by student tuition. Vocational centers are under local
school district authority, and each program area receives funds
based on a program cost factor that is plugged into a formula (cost

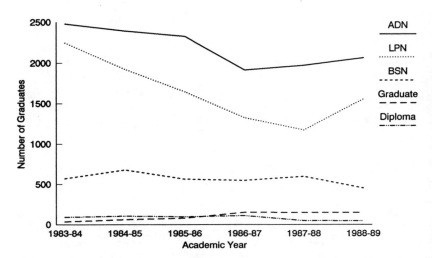

Figure 5.2. Number and Type of Graduates from Florida Nursing Programs: Academic Years 1983-1984 to 1988-1989
SOURCE: Florida Board of Nursing.

factor of 1.186 × the base student allocation × the number of hours in the program ÷ 900). In addition, school districts are required by law to charge tuition of 22.3 cents per class hour.

The availability of scholarships and loans for nursing students to finance their education is vital to nursing education. In education as a whole, including nursing, there has been a shift from scholarship aid to loan programs. This shift has increased the financial burden for nursing students because the relatively low salaries of nurses make loan repayment more difficult. Federal financial assistance for nursing students has shown a steady decline since 1979 ("As the Shortage Takes Its Toll," 1987). Most recently, the 1988 Health Omnibus Education Program Extension provides an additional $75 million for financial aid—a significant increase in federal funding for minority and disadvantaged individuals and for undergraduate, geriatric, and advanced nursing education.

In Florida, lack of state data on financial aid for nursing students hinders compilation of accurate figures on the numbers of nursing students who receive state and/or federal aid. The 1989 Florida legislature, however, created the Nursing Student Loan Forgiveness

Program to enable LPNs and RNs to retire designated percentages of the loan principal and accrued interest after working one year (25%), three years (50%), or four years (100%) in a nursing home or hospital located in the State of Florida. Funding for this program is provided by $5 annual assessment fees on nursing licenses. Employers must contribute matching funds for employees to participate in this program. While this additional money is welcomed, additional scholarships are needed to encourage bright and deserving students to enroll in nursing education programs.

Health care facilities have been important sources of financial assistance to nursing students in the past. Hospitals and nursing homes are providing nursing student scholarships, loan forgiveness programs, and employee tuition reimbursement programs. In addition, 95% of the participating nursing education programs reported that local health care and civic organizations provided nursing scholarships to their students. The 223 nursing scholarships identified in this study represent more than $525,000 in annual financial assistance to nursing students.

STUDENT RECRUITMENT

The nursing shortage and the decreases in nursing school enrollments indicate an urgent need to recruit individuals into the nursing profession. National demographic trends indicate that the number of minority and immigrant students entering the educational system is rising. While Florida statistics (Table 5.1) indicate higher percentages of males and minorities than national statistics, few gains were made in the enrollments of minorities in Florida during the early 1980s. Notable improvement was evident in the number of Hispanics completing nursing programs.

Schools of nursing need aggressive recruitment and marketing plans to attract enough applicants into nursing (Bliesmer & Eggenberger, 1989; Rosenfeld, 1988b). Respondents to the HCCCB study were asked to identify the effectiveness of a variety of recruitment strategies. Word of mouth, alumni referrals, and high school career days were ranked as the most effective recruitment strategies. In addition, associate and baccalaureate programs ranked mailing brochures and pamphlets and campus visits as effective. In contrast, LPN programs rated local advertising in newspapers and radios

TABLE 5.1 Percentage Comparison of Male and Minority Enrollments and Graduations in Florida and Nationally, 1985

Programs	Number	Enrollments			Graduations		
		Male	Black	Hispanic	Male	Black	Hispanic
LPN:							
national	851	5.6	16.9	3.8	4.8	13.6	3.1
Florida	26	7.2	21.6	4.2	6.4	18.7	3.9
A.D.N.:							
national	643	6.7	8.5	2.5	6.8	6.9	3.1
Florida	19	16.2	11.8	6.2	5.5	7.3	4.0
Diploma:							
national	203	4.8	6.8	1.8	3.5	4.2	1.7
Florida	1	7.9	21.8	21.8	7.3	13.6	33.6
B.S.N.:							
national	382	2.4	4.5	1.3	4.3	5.4	2.3
Florida	9	3.4	7.6	6.3	3.8	5.4	5.6

SOURCE: Based on data from the National League for Nursing (1987).

highly. Billboard advertising and nurse recruitment centers were judged to be the least effective strategies (Table 5.2).

Recruitment of nontraditional students is one strategy for increasing enrollments. Programs were asked to indicate whether they increased recruitment efforts for the nontraditional student populations such as males, older students (above 35 years), second-degree students, and ethnic minorities. Increased efforts to recruit males were reported by 81% of the LPN programs, 72% of the A.D.N. programs, and 73% of the B.S.N. programs; while 56% of the LPN programs, 44% of the A.D.N. programs, and 82% of the B.S.N. programs had increased efforts to recruit older students. Increased efforts were reported for recruitment of students with B.S. degrees by 33% of the A.D.N. programs and 63% of the B.S.N. programs; while 68% of LPN programs, 94% of A.D.N. programs, and 82% of B.S.N. programs reported more recruitment efforts directed toward ethnic minorities.

Increased recruitment expenses were reported by 31% of the LPN programs, 47% of the A.D.N. programs, and 73% of the B.S.N. programs. Recruitment expenses ranged from a low of $100 in several programs to a high of $94,494 in one A.D.N. program. Mean recruitment expenses were $20,494 for the 22 programs reporting recruitment expenses. Four programs indicated that student recruitment was a part of faculty regular assignments, and three programs indicated

TABLE 5.2 Effectiveness of Recruitment Strategies by Program

Strategies	Total (N = 32)	Rank Order by Program		
		LPN (N = 9)	A.D.N. (N = 15)	B.S.N. (N = 8)
Nurse recruiter	13	15	12	8
Health job fairs	8	7	9	9
High school career days	5	5	6	6
Junior/middle school career days	9	10	3	10
Word of mouth	1	1	1	1
Alumni referral	2	3	2	3
Direct phone contact	6	5	7	5
Campus visits	5	9	4	3
Campus orientation programs	10	14	8	7
Nurse recruitment centers	16	16	16	14
Local educational outreach	11	11	11	11
Billboard advertising	15	12	15	15
Newspaper advertising	7	1	9	13
Radio advertising	12	4	13	16
TV advertising	14	12	14	12
Mailing brochures/pamphlets	3	8	5	1

the parent institution assumed primary responsibilities for student recruitment.

STUDENT RETENTION

Nationally, nursing has a strong retention rate when compared with general attrition rates among students at institutions of higher learning. National statistics from NLN indicate retention rates have remained almost unchanged since 1983; however, 50% of nursing programs claim they have difficulty retaining students. Rosenfeld (1988a) reports that national retention rates vary from 88% in public three-year B.S.N. programs to 70% in public diploma programs. In general, public institutions report higher retention rates than private institutions.

Respondents to the nursing education study were asked to provide attrition rates for the past three years. Attrition rates in Florida's LPN programs decreased from 37% to 34.5% during this time, while the attrition rates in A.D.N. programs and B.S.N. programs were smaller and have decreased. A.D.N. programs reported

TABLE 5.3 Reasons for Student Withdrawal by Program

| Reasons for Withdrawing | Total | Ranking by Program | | |
		LPN	A.D.N.	B.S.N.
Family relocation	8	6	9	7
Family obligations	4	3	3	9
Personal problems	1	1	1	2
Financial difficulties	3	4	3	3
Academic difficulties	2	2	2	1
Scheduling of classes	9	8	8	8
Inflexible work schedule	5	5	5	4
Inability to find a job	10	9	11	10
Transportation difficulties	7	7	6	6
No reason given	11	11	10	11
Didn't like nursing	6	10	7	5

1989 attrition rates of 27.6%, a decrease from the 1987 rate of 30.9%. B.S.N. attrition rates fell from 12.9% in 1987 to 8.5% in 1989.

The education questionnaire asked nursing directors and deans to rank the reasons students give for withdrawing from school. Table 5.3 indicates that personal problems, academic difficulties, and financial difficulties are the top three reasons students give for withdrawing from nursing programs in Florida.

Of the nursing programs participating in the nursing education study, 69% indicated that their use of retention strategies has increased in the past three years. The cost of retention strategies varied from a low of $125 in one A.D.N. program to a high of $44,531 in a B.S.N. program. Mean retention costs for the 13 programs reporting expenses was $18,831. Several programs reported that they did not have a separate budget for retention activities but indicated that person-hours and resources were expended on student retention activities. Forty programs reported student retention was considered a part of regular faculty work load. Others stated student retention was a collegewide activity with no specific resources allocated to the nursing budget.

The five most effective retention strategies reported by respondents were learning and academic support, financial aid packages, academic advising, tutors, and early warning and prediction programs (Table 5.4). These strategies are consistent with those recommended by Allen, Nunley, and Scott-Warner (1988). Unlike Allen

TABLE 5.4 Effectiveness of Retention Strategies by Program

Retention Strategies	Total	Ranking by Program		
		LPN	A.D.N.	B.S.N.
Remedial course work	7	4	10	10
Peer counseling	9	11	8	7
Peer/faculty tutors	4	5	5	5
Academic advising	3	6	4	1
Financial aid packages	2	1	2	2
Early warning and prediction	5	3	7	3
Exit interviews	10	10	11	10
Ethnic-oriented extracurricular and cultural activities	15	12	14	13
Faculty, staff, and curricular development	8	7	6	6
Learning and academic support	1	2	1	3
Orientation	6	8	3	8
Policy changes such as in grading	11	9	12	15
Increasing minority faculty	14	13	15	12
Reduced course loads	12	14	8	9
Preceptorships	13	15	13	13

et al., however, greater availability of minority faculty and cultural activities were not perceived by respondents in this study to be effective retention strategies.

ARTICULATION AND EDUCATIONAL MOBILITY

Educational mobility has long been a goal of Florida's educational leaders. Career mobility for returning RNs and LPNs is facilitated through articulation and career ladder programs.

Articulation is the process of coordinating programs so that unnecessary duplication or gaps in students' learning are avoided as students progress among institutions and programs. Florida has addressed the issue of articulation at the state level through the Statewide Course Numbering System and the Articulation Coordinating Committee. This system facilitates the transfer of academic credit among public institutions in Florida. A Nursing Coordination Task Force was appointed in 1984 to develop an articulation plan in two areas—one to address articulation at the diploma, associate, and baccalaureate levels and another at the licensed practical nurse to associate degree levels. One articulation project was funded by the

Trust Fund for Postsecondary Cooperation. The project established a process for student articulation in nursing between Sarasota Vocational-Technical Center, Manatee Vocational-Technical Center, Manatee Community College, and the University of South Florida.

Four other B.S.N. programs surveyed in this study indicated they had written articulation agreements with local community colleges. The purpose of these agreements is to facilitate the entrance of A.D.N. graduates into the B.S.N. programs. Most of these agreements address the transfer of required prerequisite general education courses rather than nursing courses.

Career ladder programs are available in all A.D.N. programs and in all but one B.S.N. program responding to the HCCCB nursing education survey. The career ladder concept allows students to progress from practical nursing programs to associate degree and on to baccalaureate degree programs. Of the B.S.N. programs participating in the HCCCB study, only one had an RN track that was completely separate from the generic program. Other programs either integrated the RNs into their basic, generic programs or allowed the RNs to take some but not all of the nursing courses with generic students. Most A.D.N. programs allowed LPNs to take some but not all of the nursing courses with generic A.D.N. students. Some A.D.N. programs had separate programs for LPNs while others integrated the LPN into the generic program.

All of the A.D.N. programs in this study indicated they provided advanced placement for LPNs while five reported advanced placement opportunities for paramedics and military medics. Only one program allowed advanced placement for nursing assistants, EMTs, RNs with diplomas, registered respiratory therapists, and OR technicians. Three of the B.S.N. programs allowed advanced placement for LPNs and four allowed advanced placement for students with a B.S. in another discipline. Only one B.S.N. program allowed advanced placement for EMTs, paramedics, military medics, or physician assistants.

Validation of prior nursing experience is a vital part of the career ladder concept. Duplication of courses and credit prolongs the educational process and leads to increased cost for students. A variety of methods for granting credit were reported by the nursing programs participating in this study (Table 5.5). In baccalaureate programs, course-to-course transfer of nonnursing courses and standardized examinations for nursing course credits were the most frequently

TABLE 5.5 Methods of Granting Credit by Program

Methods	B.S.N. Programs		A.D.N. Programs	
	Number	Percentage	Number	Percentage
Course-to-course transfer credit of nonnursing courses	10	91	11	61
Course-to-course transfer credit of nursing courses	4	36	7	33
Teacher-made advanced placement exams for course credit	4	36	9	50
Standardized advanced placement exams for course credit	10	91	2	11
Teacher-made assessment exams for diagnostic purposes	2	18	3	17
Standardized assessment exams for diagnostic purposes	2	18	1	11
Performance-based examinations	4	36	4	22
Student portfolios	3	27	2	11

used methods. Associate degree programs were more likely to use teacher-made examinations to award course credit.

Another important component in successful career ladder programs is flexible class scheduling. Many LPNs and RNs returning to school for additional degrees are older and have children and jobs. Nursing programs were asked to indicate the percentage of courses available at night and on weekends for career ladder students. B.S.N. programs indicated 49.1%, and A.D.N. programs indicated 13.5%, of the career ladder courses were available at night and on weekends.

Issues and Findings

PERSONNEL ISSUES

In May 1987, there were 96,185 licensed RNs in Florida. More than 75,000, or 78%, were active in nursing, with 61.3% working on a full-time basis and 17% working on a part-time basis. Of the 18,905 LPNs in Florida, 15,652 (62.8%) were practicing nursing—11,984 full-time and 3,668 part-time.

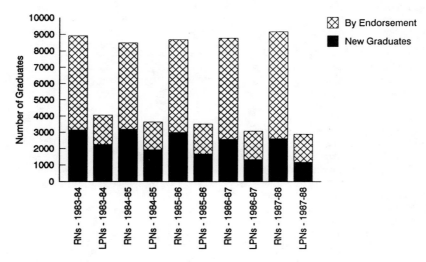

Figure 5.3. Supply of New Nurses in Florida: 1983 to 1988
SOURCE: Florida Board of Nursing.

Two personnel supply issues have emerged from this study: the low proportion of newly licensed nurses prepared by Florida's educational system and the unbalanced proportion of RNs prepared with associate, baccalaureate, and graduate degrees.

Approximately 9,000 new RNs are licensed in Florida each year. The majority (61%) of these nurses are not prepared by Florida's educational system but are licensed RNs who have moved from other states to Florida. The percentage (39%) of newly licensed RNs prepared by Florida's educational programs has declined during the past three years. Figure 5.3 provides data comparing the numbers of new graduates with nurses licensed by endorsement.

Florida, unlike some states, is fortunate in that the state attracts large numbers of licensed nurses from other parts of the country. There is reason to question whether this trend will continue in the future. Florida hospitals have traditionally recruited in the northeastern part of the country. As salaries in the Northeast continue to rise dramatically ("New Salary Wars Promise," 1988; "Pennsylvania RNs' Salary Goals," 1988), the inability of Florida hospitals to match these salaries may limit the influx of licensed nurses from other parts of the United States.

A second nurse supply problem is the proportion of associate-, baccalaureate-, and graduate-prepared nurses in Florida. Of the RNs practicing in Florida, only 25.7% have baccalaureate degrees while 5.7% have master's degrees and 0.5% doctorates (Florida State Board of Nursing, 1988). These percentages do not distinguish between nursing and nonnursing degrees. Of the RNs licensed in 1988, 80.4% were prepared in associate degree programs and 17.7% in baccalaureate programs. The number of nurses prepared at the graduate level has shown improvement as the number of master's and doctoral programs have increased. In 1989, 144 nurses received master's degrees in nursing and 7 received doctorates in nursing (Figure 5.2).

U.S. DHHS (1988) projections indicate Florida will increasingly have a surplus of associate degree nurses and a deficit of nurses with baccalaureate and graduate degrees. Florida currently has no statewide educational policy or formula to meet current or future demands for various categories of licensed nurses. The number of nurses with baccalaureate and graduate degrees in Florida must continually be monitored, and increased support must be given to those programs to ensure that Florida has adequate numbers of nurses prepared at appropriate levels of education.

CONCERNS OF DEANS AND DIRECTORS

The deans and directors of nursing programs who responded to this survey identified four major issues or concerns on their programs: the academic ability of students applying for admission, the high clinical student-faculty ratios, inadequate financial support, and noncompetitive faculty salaries. The remainder of this chapter will address these concerns.

Student ability. Lowering admission standards is one method to maintain numbers of admissions and enrollments in nursing programs. The nursing education study asked participating programs to indicate changes made in program admission requirements for the past three years. Only four programs indicated a decrease in the required number of prerequisite courses. No programs reported lower SAT/ACT or GPA admission requirements. Only one program lowered the GPA retention requirement. Some programs indicated that they had not lowered standards but were accepting every student that met the admission requirements in order to maintain enrollments. Several B.S.N. programs stated that the demand for admission continued to exceed availability and that student enrollment could be increased if adequate funding for additional faculty was provided.

Nationally, the rising failure rates on national state board examinations may reflect declining admission standards (Rosenfeld, 1988b). The national failure rate for first-time U.S.-educated nurses on the July 1988 RN licensure examination reached a record high of 16.4%, some 60% higher than the 10% failure rate recorded in 1983 (U.S. DHHS, 1988). Leaders of the Council of State Boards attribute two factors to the increased failure rate: a slightly higher passing standard combined with a decline in students' capabilities ("State Board Failure Rate," 1988).

Florida statistics demonstrate that the failure rate has increased during the past five years from 7% in 1983-1984 to 19% in 1988-1989. The failure rate on the LPN board examinations has increased from 6% in 1983-1984 to 9% in 1987-1988. Table 5.6 presents the percentages and numbers of RNs who passed the RN state board examinations in the United States and Florida between 1983 and 1989. The higher failure rates on RN and LPN examinations directly affect the adequacy of nurse staffing for those health institutions hiring new graduates. When a nurse fails the licensure examination, he or she can no longer work as a graduate nurse and must assume a position as a nonlicensed health care worker until he or she has successfully passed the next licensure examination. The National Council of State Boards of Nursing has received requests from some states to increase the frequency of administering the NCLEX test to put those failing the exam back into the work force more quickly ("State Board Failure . . . ," 1988).

The data collected in this study indicate generally that admission and retention criteria in Florida's nursing programs have not been lowered in recent years. Increased use of tutorial and remedial activities and a higher state board failure rate, however, may indirectly indicate some lowering of standards. Faculty should continue to monitor the quality of students being admitted and not lower standards simply to maintain enrollments.

Clinical ratios. The maximum clinical student-faculty ratio allowed by the Florida Board of Nursing is 12:1. This ratio, one of the top concerns of deans and directors, was thought by some respondents to be unsafe in some clinical areas. Comments indicated that

TABLE 5.6 RN State Board Passage Rates by Type of Program, 1983-1988

Test Dates	National %	Florida %	B.S.N. %	B.S.N. N	Florida Programs A.D.N. %	A.D.N. N	Diploma %	Diploma N
1983:								
July	90	94	89	255	94	1583	89	55
1984:								
February	90	91	91	189	91	632	93	30
July	89	91	82	299	92	1650	89	50
1985:								
February	89	91	91	66	92	693	77	49
July	91	91	89	356	92	1568	80	59
1986:								
February	90	89	82	93	90	714	93	42
July	92	92	87	405	94	1505	94	62
1987:								
February	89	87	84	90	94	622	94	44
July	91	89	86	368	90	1192	90	27
1988:								
February	87	87	83	93	88	565	97	30
July	85	84	84	326	83	1072	90	18
1989:								
February	85	81	84	74	81	563	96	25
July	86.5	87	89	349	86	1050	93.5	29

SOURCE: Florida State Board of Nursing and "State Board Failure Rate" (1988).

two factors—increased patient acuity and lower student abilities—have contributed to this growing concern. This study did not attempt to address the most effective student-faculty ratios in various clinical settings. Additional research is needed to provide an empirical basis for determining appropriate staffing requirements for faculty.

Financial support. Financial support for nursing education continues to be an issue. Inadequate funds for faculty salaries and resources (equipment, books, computers) were reported by deans and directors, with 70% of associate degree programs reporting that faculty salaries were $2,000-$12,000 lower than surrounding health care facilities' salaries. Average mean faculty salaries in Florida do not appear to differ greatly from nationally reported salaries. Florida salaries, however, do not reflect different levels of academic preparation (Table 5.7).

TABLE 5.7 Mean Annual Faculty Salaries by Program

Type of Program	1988-1989 Florida Salaries (in dollars)		1986-1987 National Salaries (in dollars)	
	Minimum	Maximum	Minimum	Maximum
LPN:*				
Instructor	20,000	46,000	14,059	25,970
A.D.N.:**				
instructor	18,200	44,304	10,000	42,000
assistant professor	18,800	45,523	12,700	40,500
associate professor	20,600	43,120	17,000	45,900
professor	30,200	39,100	15,600	55,200
B.S.N.:***				
instructor	18,000	25,358	NA	NA
assistant professor	23,000	30,570	NA	NA
associate professor	30,000	39,510	NA	NA
professor	NA	NA	NA	NA
BSN and graduate:***				
instructor	24,000	36,720	10,400	32,200
assistant professor	24,300	44,354	18,000	41,300
associate professor	29,000	54,600	14,900	52,700
professor	43,000	60,214	14,200	66,400

SOURCE: Based on data from the National League for Nursing (1987).
*Twelve-month appointment only.
**Nine- to ten-month academic appointment only. Academic ranks or equivalents used.
***Nine- to ten-month academic appointment only.

Of the associate degree nursing programs in Florida, 72% require faculty to have a master's degree in nursing or a related discipline. Nurses with master's degrees are generally used as middle managers (head nurses) or clinical specialists in hospitals. The Cole Nurse Compensation Study (Cole & Sizing, 1988) indicates nurses in these positions earn $31,600-$35,200 annually. Entry-level salaries for faculty in nursing programs are significantly less than salaries available in the health care industry.

A.D.N. programs appear to be having the most difficulty with faculty vacancies. Only three A.D.N. programs reported having no unfilled faculty positions for the 1989-1990 academic year. A.D.N. programs reported that the most difficult positions to fill were in medical-surgical, maternity, and pediatric nursing. Noncompetitive salaries and increased work loads are likely to contribute to higher faculty vacancies.

Four B.S.N. programs (36%) responding to this study indicated that they had no unfilled faculty positions for the 1989-1990 academic year. The most critical need for faculty in B.S.N. programs was in medical-surgical nursing. Unfilled positions in maternity nursing, in foundations, in nursing research, and for nurse practitioners were also reported by three programs.

Overall, respondents reported that recruiting qualified faculty for medical-surgical nursing positions was the most difficult. Pediatrics and maternity nursing faculty were also reported to be difficult positions in terms of recruitment.

Use of part-time faculty and adjunct faculty are two strategies for dealing with noncompetitive salaries and increased work loads, and 45% of associate degree programs and 30% of baccalaureate programs indicated their use of part-time faculty had increased since 1986. Use of faculty with adjunct or joint appointments, however, is not prevalent in many nursing programs, especially associate degree programs.

Currently, health care agencies provide financial assistance to nursing programs with adjunct and/or joint faculty appointments. Eighteen nursing programs reported having 154 adjunct faculty positions. Most of these positions were initiated by the educational institution. Only 5 nursing programs out of 17 reported use of faculty joint appointments; these faculty provide predetermined services to both institutions and may be financially supported by the educational institution, the health care agency, or both. Three programs reported that local health care agencies support one or more of their joint appointment faculty positions. Most of these positions are currently financed by the educational institution.

The 1989 Florida legislature created two opportunities for health care institutions to become more involved in providing financial support for nursing education. The first legislative action established the nursing Education Challenge Grant Fund for Community Colleges. This fund matches private contributions with state funding and supports student enrollments in nursing and allied health programs in Florida community colleges. These funds may be used for faculty salaries and expenses, books, equipment, recruiting efforts, tuition, hospital internships, and in-kind contributions. Universities are not eligible for these funds. Approximately $800,000 in state general revenue funds were authorized for the 23 matches in 1990.

The second legislative action removed regulatory barriers to hospitals increasing their financial involvement in health education. This law provides that direct costs arising from assistance provided to expand or supplement the curriculum for nurses or other health professionals, not including physicians, be considered a pass-through for Health Care Cost Containment Board purposes. The financial assistance includes but is not limited to the direct cost of community college, university, or vocational training school faculty salaries and expenses, books, equipment, recruiting efforts, tuition assistance, hospital internships, and in-kind contributions.

Conclusion

Professional nursing is practiced in complex and dynamic health care settings. Today's health care requires critical thinking, problem-solving, and management skills in nurses. Contemporary nursing practice demands a knowledge of chemistry, physiology, mathematics, and language. It is essential that nursing education and practice continue to be of high quality and not be compromised by the nursing shortage in Florida.

Nursing education must be responsive to the dramatic changes occurring in the health care industry by emphasizing critical thinking, problem solving, computer literacy, personnel and fiscal management, technology, critical care, and gerontological nursing. It is the responsibility of the Florida Board of Nursing to ensure that curricula are relevant to contemporary and future nursing practice. Furthermore, collaborative activity between nursing service and nursing education is needed to ensure that nursing education reflects current nursing practice, to facilitate faculty research and practice opportunities, to create adjunct and joint faculty positions, to investigate the appropriate student/faculty ratios in various clinical settings, and to prepare students in a variety of practice settings.

Florida is experiencing a critical shortage of professional nurses. Current manpower projections indicate that the shortage is long term and will worsen, especially for nurses with baccalaureate and graduate degrees. Greater proportions of registered nurses who are licensed each year in Florida should be prepared by Florida's educational system to meet the demands for nurses and limit Florida's dependency on other states. Those schools of professional nursing with student demand and adequate classroom and clinical facilities should increase enrollments and should be provided with funding to do so. Availability of and access to baccalaureate and graduate education should be increased to provide adequate numbers of nurse managers, faculty, clinical specialists, and administrators.

The decreased recruitment pool of 18- to 24-year-old students will require nursing to attract a substantial number of minority and nontraditional students. To meet the needs of a diverse student population and accommodate part-time students, nursing education programs will have to increase educational mobility with maximum transfer of credit and offer flexible scheduling, including a mixture of day, evening, weekend, and summer classes. Flexibility in scheduling will be enhanced if incentive funding is provided to programs offering such scheduling and to faculty who teach these classes. Mobility can be facilitated by providing remedial bridge programs to upgrade basic language and mathematics skills for students with disadvantaged backgrounds. Access to career mobility programs will be enhanced by requiring a minimum of a high school diploma for all categories of health personnel (including nursing assistant categories).

Increased enrollment in nursing education programs is dependent upon the availability of qualified applicants, the number of faculty, the availability of clinical sites, and the availability of resources within the educational institution. Adequate financial support for programs and students is needed. Faculty salaries in some parts of the state are not competitive with salaries offered by local health care institutions. Current financial aid records are inadequate to assess the magnitude of the financial aid needed for nursing students. The decline in federal financial aid and the focus on nontraditional and disadvantaged students will require additional private and state resources for the recruitment and retention of these students. Currently, health care agencies have an opportunity to support nursing education through the Nursing Education Challenge Grant Fund for Community Colleges. Additional merit and need scholarships for students should be established by state, professional, philanthropic, and health care organizations. Sources of financial support such as educational scholarships, loans, and stipends need to be identified, published, and distributed by nursing programs to prospective students.

And, finally, nursing education programs, professional nurse associations, and employers should assume responsibility for socializing entering students into the profession to ensure that the nursing career choice remains a lifelong decision. These factors include socialization into the nursing role, commitment to the profession, and emphasis on the attractiveness of the profession. Nursing education programs should identify nursing students early in their educational experience and initiate activities that incorporate them into the nursing role. In addition, externship programs need to be instituted to link nursing students with excellent, highly experienced nurses who can serve as role models.

SIX

Hospital Perspectives on Nurse Employment

WILLIAM J. SEROW

MARIE E. COWART

YEN CHEN

Nationwide, and in Florida, hospitals constitute the primary locus of employment for nursing personnel. Data from the latter portion of the 1980s show that about two thirds of Florida's registered nurses (RNs) were employed in hospitals, as were more than 40% of the state's licensed practical nurses (LPNs; Florida Department of Health and Rehabilitative Services [DHRS], 1987). Speake (1990) reports on similar employment distributions in several additional states, especially with regard to RNs. Clearly, then, any consideration of the labor market for nursing personnel must include a social accounting of the conditions of their employment in hospital settings.

This chapter begins with a brief review of the characteristics of those nurses employed within the hospital industry in Florida and then reports upon the findings of our survey of these institutions with respect to the shortage of nursing personnel. In addition to reporting upon both subjective and objective measures of the overall shortage, we consider the extent of turnover among nursing personnel in the industry. The chapter reports on the degree and severity of these measures with regard to characteristics of the hospital (geographic location within Florida, type of ownership, type of care provided, size) and of nurses themselves and their employment settings (specialty, shift, season). The chapter then reviews what might be termed the *causes* of the shortage, especially with regard to trends in salary and benefit levels across the industry, and then considers what might be termed the *consequences* of the shortage, that is, the responses of the institutions themselves to actual and perceived shortage through the expenditure of funds for overtime and temporary staff as well as through longer-term strategies aimed at recruiting *and* retaining nursing personnel.

Overview of the Sample

CHARACTERISTICS OF HOSPITALS

Of the 301 hospitals listed with the Florida Health Care Cost Containment Board at the beginning of 1989, some 296 were deemed "eligible" for inclusion in our survey. Of these, responses were received from 287, or 97%. Of the 246 hospitals that reported their number of beds, about one fourth (66) had fewer than 100 beds, while slightly more than one tenth had at least 500. The mean and median number of beds was 224 and 175, respectively. Of the 282 hospitals that reported their ownership, nearly half (132) were proprietary (for profit), while some 40% (108) were nonprofit. The remaining 15% (42 facilities) were publicly owned. As would be expected, the spatial distribution of hospitals was broadly similar to that of Florida's population, with some overrepresentation in the Tallahassee, Gainesville, and Tampa areas and some underrepresentation in both the southeastern and the southwestern portions of the state as well as in greater Orlando. Nineteen of the hospitals were the sole county providers. About three fourths of the hospitals in the sample (207) were acute care, short-term facilities with the remainder scattered among long-term care, rehabilitation, psychiatric, and other specialty hospitals. Federally owned institutions were excluded, but the sample is a heterogeneous one, providing a broad perspective of the hospital employment picture.

CHARACTERISTICS OF NURSES

A slight majority of all hospital-employed RNs reported holding an associate degree, slightly more than one fourth had earned a diploma from a hospital-based RN program, and the remaining 21% reported holding one or more university degrees. It is perhaps surprising that this share is slightly less than that reported for nursing home or home health agency employed nurses (23% each). The median age of RNs employed in Florida's hospitals was 39.5 years, nearly 10 years younger than for registered nurses employed in nursing homes (48.8 years) and about the same as those employed in other institutional settings. About one third of RNs employed in hospitals fell into the age ranges of below 35, 35 to 44, and 45 and older. There is some tendency for younger nurses to be employed in larger hospitals, perhaps reflecting the location of such facilities in larger urban areas, which might be more attractive to younger persons. Finally, the median number of years employed at their current location for all RNs and LPNs was about 3.7 years, a substantially longer period than for nurses employed in nursing homes (2.6 years), in home health agencies (1.6 years), or in hospices (1.7 years).

In 1988, the average hospital employed about 165 nursing personnel (full-time equivalent) per 100 *occupied* beds; of these, about 60% were RNs, with the remainder about equally split between LPNs and nursing assistants (NAs). Over time, this ratio has risen from 162 in 1984 and 1985 to a maximum of 172 in 1987 before declining in the year prior to the survey. Reductions in staffing were observable for all three types of personnel. Hospitals in the smallest size category (fewer than 100 beds) reported substantially higher ratios (nearly 200 to 100) of personnel to occupied beds than all larger hospitals, perhaps reflecting lower occupancy rates. With the exception of the five specialty hospitals (nearly 200 FTE nursing personnel per 100 occupied beds), short-stay acute care facilities reported much higher staffing ratios than did all other types (181 and 118, respectively).

Vacancy and Turnover Rates Among Nursing Personnel in Florida Hospitals

VACANCY RATES

Vacancy rates as reported by hospitals for the year 1988 averaged 17% for RNs, 20% for LPNs, and 18% for NAs. There was considerable variation in these levels according to the size, type of ownership, and type of care provided by each hospital. The *number of beds* in a hospital was inversely related to the vacancy rate for each of the three types of nursing personnel: the larger the hospital, the

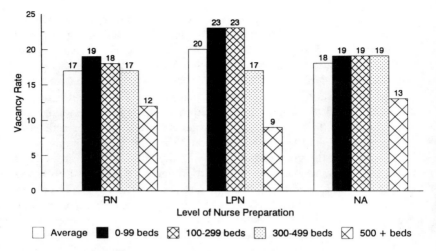

Figure 6.1. Vacancy Rates for Nursing Staff by Level of Preparation and Size of Hospital: Florida Hospitals: 1988

lower the vacancy rate. The differences were most apparent be-tween the largest size group (500 beds or more) and all smaller fa-cilities. Vacancy rates among RNs in the former were only 12%, on average, compared with levels of 17% to 19% otherwise. Similarly, vacancies accounted for 9% of budgeted LPN slots in large institu-tions versus 17% to 23% in smaller ones and for 13% of budgeted NA slots in large institutions versus 19% (see Figure 6.1).

The picture is not nearly so clear-cut with regard to *hospital owner-ship*. Vacancy rates for RNs were marginally higher in publicly owned facilities (19%) than in either not-for-profits or proprietaries (17%) but were lower for LPNs (11%, 17%, and 24%, respectively). Nonprofit in-stitutions had somewhat lower vacancy rates for NAs (14%) than did either publicly owned or profit-making hospitals (see Figure 6.2). Fi-nally, vacancy rates for both RNs and LPNs were noticeably lower in acute care, short-term stay hospitals (17% and 18%) than in other car-egiving types (25% and 33%) but were higher for nursing assistants (19% in the former, 14% in the latter). These are shown in Figure 6.3.

Among registered nurses, the survey data also provided informa-tion on vacancy rates according to the nurse's primary assignment within the hospital: intensive or coronary care units (ICU), emergency

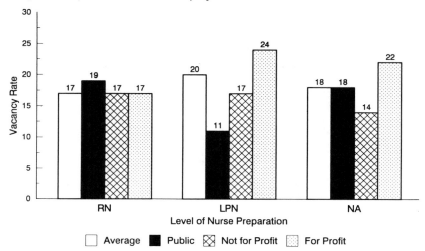

Figure 6.2. Vacancy Rates for Nursing Staff by Level of Preparation and Ownership of Hospital

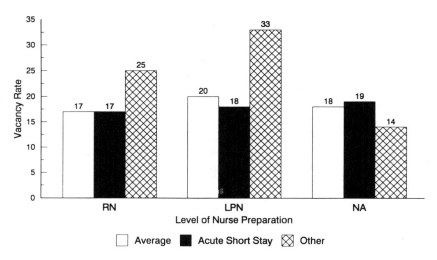

Figure 6.3. Hospital Vacancy Rates for Nursing Staff by Level of Preparation and Type of Care

rooms (ER), operating rooms (OR), and general medical-surgical assignments (MS). These are shown in Figure 6.4, arrayed by size of

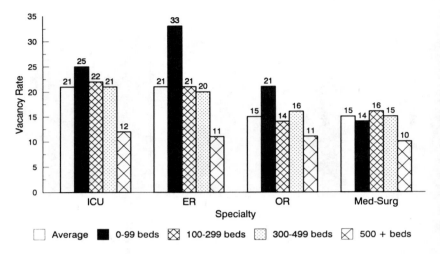

Figure 6.4. Vacancy Rates for Registered Nurses by Nursing Specialty and Size of Hospital

employing institution. Overall, vacancy rates are six percentage points higher for RN positions budgeted for ICUs and ERs (21% each) than for those located in the remaining two sectors. The overall inverse relationship between size of the hospital and the vacancy rate is evident in these data as well, as vacancies are much more uncommon in hospitals of 500 or more beds regardless of the area of assignment. Similarly, vacancy rates are at a maximum within the smallest-sized hospitals across all sectors.

In addition to these data, which might be considered "objective" measures of shortage, the survey also asked respondents to provide their assessment of the "seriousness" of the shortage in their own hospitals by means of a five-point scale in which higher scores are indicative of a higher level of concern on the part of the respondent. The results are summarized in Table 6.1.

Collectively, the degree of seriousness expressed by those responding to the survey was somewhat predictable in that shortages were perceived as most problematic for those shifts that would tend to be viewed as undesirable (evenings and nights) and for those days of the week that would tend to be viewed as undesirable (Saturday and Sunday). The fall and, particularly, the winter of the year

TABLE 6.1 Reported Seriousness of Nursing Shortages in Florida Hospitals

Specialty	Day of Week		Position		Season		Shift	
ICU: 3.5	Wednesday:	2.3	Staff:	3.2	Spring:	2.7	Day:	2.1
ER: 2.3	Saturday:	3.6	Charge:	2.4	Summer:	2.3	Evening:	3.3
OR: 2.2	Sunday:	3.5	Head Nurse:	1.6	Fall:	3.0	Night:	3.5
MS: 3.1					Winter:	3.5		

NOTE: Seriousness scale: 1 = not serious to 5 = very serious.

are times when shortages seem to be most acute, reflecting a seasonal increase in demand for hospital beds as a result of Florida's position as the winter residence of a relatively large number of persons, often elderly, from elsewhere in the United States and from Canada (Marshall & Longino, 1988). Additionally, shortages were felt to be more severe for budgeted staff rather than supervisory positions as well as for ICU and medical-surgical (MS) positions, at least partially (with respect to ICU) confirming the differential vacancy rates by assignment shown in Figure 6.4.

TURNOVER RATES

Turnover rates as reported by hospitals for the year 1988 averaged 28% for RNs, 33% for LPNs, and 37% for NAs. There was considerable variation in these levels according to the size, type of ownership, and type of care provided by each hospital, largely paralleling the results reported above for vacancy rates. The number of beds in a hospital was inversely related to the turnover rate for each of the three types of nursing personnel: the larger the hospital, the lower the turnover rate. The differences were most apparent between the largest size group (500 beds or more) and all smaller facilities, especially with regard to LPNs and NAs. Turnover rates among RNs in the former were only 18%, on average, compared with levels of 25% to 33% otherwise. Similarly, turnover amounted to 15% of budgeted LPN slots in large institutions versus 31% to 47% in smaller ones and to 21% of budgeted NA slots in large institutions versus 35% to 44% (see Figure 6.5).

The situation is also quite clear-cut with regard to hospital ownership. Turnover rates for all categories of nursing personnel were appreciably and consistently higher in profit-making facilities than in either not-for-profits or publicly owned hospitals. The margin of

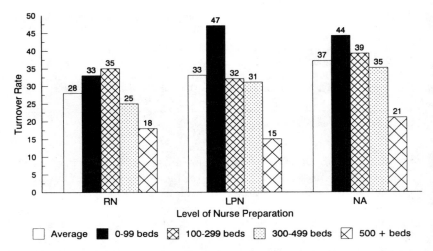

Figure 6.5. Turnover Rates for Nursing Staff by Level of Preparation and Size of Hospital

difference amounted to 5 to 10 percentage points for RNs, 11 to 15 percentage points for LPNs, and 11 or 12 percentage points for NAs. Publicly owned institutions had somewhat lower turnover rates than did not-for-profits for both RNs and LPNs, perhaps reflecting a desire among nurses employed in this portion of the industry to become vested in the public sector retirement system (see Figure 6.6).

Finally, turnover rates for all three types of nursing personnel were substantially lower in acute care, short-stay hospitals. Other caregiving types of hospitals experienced turnover rates approximately half again as great for RNs and NAs and nearly twice as much for LPNs. These are shown in Figure 6.7.

Among registered nurses, the survey data also provided information on turnover rates according to the nurse's primary assignment within the hospital; these are shown in Figure 6.8, arrayed by size of employing institution. Unlike the case of vacancy rates, where RN positions budgeted for ICUs and ERs were filled less often than those located in the remaining two sectors, turnover rates were at a minimum in the former areas. The contrast is especially striking between ICU and MS slots. The overall inverse relationship between size of the hospital and turnover rate is evident in these data as

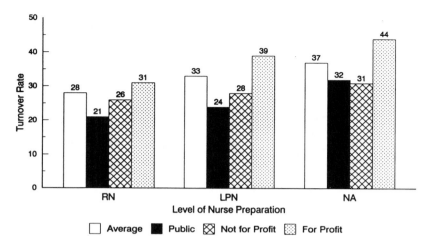

Figure 6.6. Hospital Turnover Rates for Nursing Staff by Level of Preparation

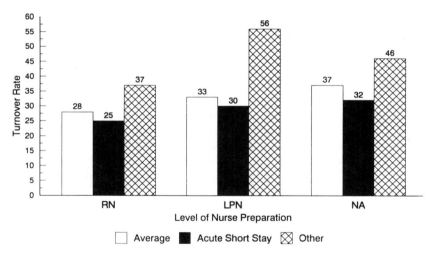

Figure 6.7. Hospital Turnover Rates for Nursing Staff by Level of Preparation and Type of Care

well, as turnover occurs at a consistently lower rate in hospitals of 500 or more beds regardless of the area of assignment. Similarly,

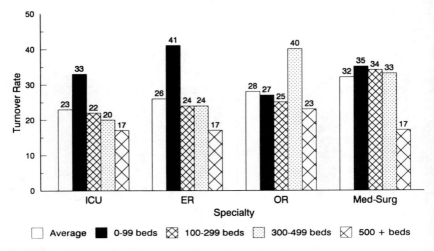

Figure 6.8. Turnover Rates for Registered Nurses by Nursing Specialty and Size of Hospital

vacancy rates are at a maximum within the smallest-sized hospitals across all sectors, with the exception of OR rates.

Causes of the Shortage

Our approach to identifying the causes of the nursing shortage will proceed along two lines. First, we shall summarize reported information relating to salary and benefit levels in an effort to suggest how comparatively low levels of each tend to make it difficult for hospitals to attract and retain nursing personnel. Second, we shall summarize the results of our regression analyses, which endeavor to uncover the impact of the hospital characteristics described previously upon vacancy, turnover, and perceived seriousness of the shortage.

SALARIES AND BENEFITS

Beginning hourly salary for registered nurses varied only very slightly according to the amount of educational preparation, with those RNs holding an A.D.N. receiving an average of $10.31, those with a hospital-based nursing school diploma an average of $10.43, and those with a B.S.N. degree some $10.60. Some variation may be observed with regard to geographic location within Florida, as pay differentials favor the large urban (and relatively high cost-of-living) areas in southeastern Florida. If we consider the modal category of nurse preparation (A.D.N. degree), variation in starting salary is evident according to ownership, type of care provided, and size of the hospital.

Average starting salaries for nurses with this type of preparation are highest among not-for-profits ($10.38), followed closely by proprietaries ($10.21) and public institutions ($10.08). The average starting salary for those nurses employed in short-stay, acute care hospitals was $10.30 per hour, some 10 cents per hour less than that offered nurses employed by other types of hospitals. Overall, the median beginning salary for this type of nurse was $10.47; hospitals with fewer than 100 beds and with 100 to 299 beds offered starting salaries below this level ($10.34 and $10.46, respectively). The highest starting salary was offered by those institutions with between 300 and 500 beds ($10.76 per hour), while those with more than 500 beds were only marginally above the median at $10.50 per hour.

Average starting salaries for LPNs and NAs were $7.20 and $4.64, respectively; again, geographic variation provided higher salary levels in the southeastern quadrant of the state. With regard to the size of the employing hospital, a pattern identical to that for RNs may be found in that the highest salaries are paid by hospitals with 300 to 500 beds and the lowest by the smallest hospitals.

The median increase in starting salary during the past year was 7.7% for RNs, 7.3% for LPNs, and 5.8% for NAs. These varied systematically only according to ownership and were quite consistent in that proprietaries always had provided the greatest relative increase over the year, and publicly owned hospitals, the lowest. There was very little difference in the value of the fringe benefit package (expressed as a percentage of salary); for each of the three categories of nursing personnel, the employing hospital viewed the package as representing about one fourth of salary. These salary and benefit data are summarized in Table 6.2.

REGRESSION ANALYSES

In an effort to determine the degree of interaction among those variables that are related to the nursing shortage and to provide

TABLE 6.2 Summary Salary and Fringe Benefit Data for Florida
Hospitals (in dollars)

		RNs			LPN	NA
	Total	A.D.N	Diploma	B.S.N.		
Mean hourly starting salary:						
total		10.31	10.43	10.60	7.20	4.64
public		10.08				
not for profit		10.38				
proprietary		10.21				
acute short stay		10.30				
other		10.40				
Median hourly starting salary:						
total	10.47				7.14	4.67
0-99 beds	10.34				6.95	4.42
100-299 beds	10.46				7.13	4.68
300-499 beds	10.76				7.40	5.01
500+ beds	10.50				7.13	4.66
Median increase in starting salary:						
total	(7.7%)				(7.3%)	(5.8%)
public	(5.7%)				(4.9%)	(4.6%)
not for profit	(7.3%)				(6.6%)	(5.7%)
proprietary	(9.1%)				(9.0%)	(6.4%)
Median value of fringe benefits						
(percentage of salary)	(25.2%)				(25.8%)	(26.1%)

some initial insights into their relationship with response mechanisms, we have conducted multiple regression analyses of vacancy and turnover rates for all RNs, RNs by assignment (ICU, ER, OR, MS), all LPNs, and all NAs. These regressions were estimated using dummy variables for geographic location (Florida Department of Health and Rehabilitative Services district) and ownership type as well as number of beds and whether the institution was the sole hospital in its county. These results are displayed in Tables 6.3 and 6.4.

Statistically significant equations emerge for RN vacancy rates in ICU, ER, and MS settings as well as among all LPNs. Geographic location is quite important, and all statistically significant coefficients indicate rates lower than that of the reference area, District 11 (Miami). Ownership is also important and, in general, both public and not-for-profit facilities experience lower rates than do those operated for profit. For ICU and ER settings, an institution that is the

TABLE 6.3 Summary of Regressions of FTE Turnover and Vacancy Rates by Department: Florida Hospitals, 1988

Independent Variable	Total Vacancy	Total Turnover	ICU Vacancy	ER Vacancy	OR Vacancy	MS Vacancy	ICU Turnover	ER Turnover	OR Turnover	MS Turnover
Region 1	-.184***	-.036	-.249**	.046	-.028	-.137#	.017	.013	-.121	-.083
Region 2	-.135#	.005	-.214**	-.038	-.045	-.007	-.034	.022	-.077	-.021
Region 3	-.077	.078	-.179***	-.027	-.021	.023	-.125	-.086	.050	-.037
Region 4	-.105	.052	-.235**	-.067	-.207#	-.075	-.061	-.049	-.138	-.084
Region 5	-.011	.069	-.208***	.006	.025	-.011	.047	-.145	-.025	-.037
Region 6	-.176***	.115	-.173#	.033	-.189#	-.086	.121	.024	-.096	.050
Region 7	-.111	.013	-.216**	-.070	-.124	-.085	.067	-.040	-.151	-.048
Region 8	-.168***	.006	-.258*	-.103	-.091	-.066	-.073	-.095	-.106	-.071
Region 9	-.153#	.002	-.163#	-.116	-.157	-.084	.021	-.142	-.156#	-.065
Region 10	-.048	-.002	-.127	.084	-.130	.061	-.025	-.093	-.090	-.056
Public	-.064	-.106	-.028	-.104	-.115	-.239**	.043	-.152#	-.037	-.185***
Not for profit	-.077	-.083	-.204***	-.194#	-.205***	-.227**	.016	-.110	-.212***	-.216**
Sole co-county provider	.060	-.033	.138#	.191***	.057	-.012	.021***	.020	-.033	.071
Number of beds	-.116#	-.144***	-.149***	-.177#	-.109	-.041	-.174***	-.184#	.053	-.125#
R-square adjusted	.028	.006	.107	.081	.035	.067	.032	0	.009	.025
F	1.5	1.1	2.6	1.8	1.3	2.1	1.4	0.9	1.1	1.4
Significance	NS	NS	<.01	<.05	NS	<.05	NS	NS	NS	NS

NOTE: Data shown are standardized (beta) regression coefficients. Values for regions are relative to the omitted category, region 11. Values for ownership are relative to the omitted category, for profit.

*p < .001; **p < .01; ***p < .05; #p < .10.

TABLE 6.4 Summary of Regressions of FTE Turnover and Vacancy Rates by Position: Florida Hospitals, 1988

Independent Variable	RNs Vacancy	RNs Turnover	LPNs Vacancy	LPNs Turnover	NAs Vacancy	NAs Turnover	Temporary Staff Expenditure per Bed
Region 1	-.180***	-.036	-.241**	-.059	.122	-.079	-.213***
Region 2	-.172***	-.011	-.310**	-.113	-.048	.275*	-.101
Region 3	-.066	.131#	-.315**	.059	-.065	.004	-.030
Region 4	-.189***	.025	-.299**	-.040	-.106	.054	-.050
Region 5	-.126	-.000	-.292**	-.063	-.063	.094	-.014
Region 6	-.183***	.121	-.205#	-.052	-.106	.095	-.098
Region 7	-.170***	-.026	-.222***	.020	-.106	.076	.087
Region 8	-.185***	.028	-.281**	-.081	-.138	.025	-.101
Region 9	-.173***	.032	-.271***	-.127	-.110	.116	.254**
Region 10	-.123	-.052	-.113	-.092	-.082	.152#	-.015
Public	.086	-.135***	-.167***	-.112	-.070	-.125	-.154#
Not for profit	.030	-.115#	-.081	-.135#	-.243***	-.116	-.091
Sole co-county provider	.083	-.045	.007	-.041	.087	-.095	.004
Number of beds	-.184***	-.154***	-.237**	-.203**	-.025	-.187***	-.045
less than 100 beds							-.298***
100-299 beds							-.152
300-499 beds							-.151
Total vacancy rate							.136#
Total turnover rate							-.178***
R-square adjusted	.027	.041	.138	.051	0	.081	.189
F	1.5	1.8	2.8	1.8	0.9	2.2	2.9
Significance	NS	<.05	<.001	<.05	NS	<.01	<.001

NOTE: Data shown are standardized (beta) regression coefficients. Values for regions are relative to the omitted category, region 11. Values for ownership are relative to the omitted category, for profit. Values for size in expenditures for temporary staff per bed are relative to the omitted category, more than 500.
*p < .001; **p < .01; ***p < .05; #p < .10.

sole county provider is apt to experience higher vacancy rates than an otherwise identical institution that is not. This suggests a greater problem in rural localities, which are those most likely to have a single institution. Size of the institution is also an important determinant and, other things being equal, vacancy is less problematic among larger institutions.

The only significant equations for turnover rates are those estimated for all RNs, all LPNs, and all NAs. These equations are largely a function of bed size and ownership, which operate in the same manner as for vacancy rates.

An additional set of regressions were estimated for the perceived seriousness of the shortage, according to nursing assignment (ICU, ER, OR, MS), shift, day of the week, and season of the year. The dependent variables used for this analysis include the regional and ownership dummies as well as salary and benefit measures. The results of this analysis are presented in Table 6.5.

The only statistically significant equations pertain to seriousness during the winter months and on Saturday. Seriousness during the winter is more of a problem in the reference area (District 11) than elsewhere, with significantly lower perceptions of seriousness in the northern and east-central regions of the state, which host comparatively few "snowbirds." Larger hospitals and those with lower starting salaries (and, by extension, lower salary levels in general) also perceive this problem to be more serious. Seriousness of the shortage for Saturday shifts is also more pronounced in District 11 than elsewhere, with significantly lower degrees of this perception in the Gainesville, Jacksonville, Tampa, Fort Myers, and West Palm Beach areas. Shortages on this day are also perceived as being more problematic within the proprietary segment of the industry, especially relative to not-for-profits.

Impacts of the Shortage

There are a variety of strategies that hospitals employ to cope with problems of vacancy and turnover among nursing personnel. Some of these might be termed *procedural* and would include reactions, such as closing beds, that deviate from established standards, especially with regard to the timing of admissions and medical procedures. A second type of strategy might be termed *financial* and

TABLE 6.5 Summary of Regressions of Perceived Seriousness by Assignment and Shift

Independent Variable	Medical-Surgical	ICU	ER	OR	Staff	Fall	Winter	Saturday	Sunday	Evening	Night
Region 1	.062	-.193	-.105	-.051	-.150	-.299**	-.169#	-.157#	-.130	-.112	-.196#
Region 2	.150	-.184#	-.168	.078	.091	-.236***	-.154	-.161	-.096	.064	-.209***
Region 3	-.191#	-.321***	-.204	-.122	-.048	-.337**	-.203***	-.223***	-.188#	-.055	-.146
Region 4	-.059	-.114	-.163	-.075	-.031	-.267***	-.281**	-.196#	-.158	.030	-.117
Region 5	.045	-.211	-.397**	-.256***	.037	-.238***	.018	-.014	.023	.089	-.104
Region 6	-.075	-.169	-.285***	-.178	-.121	-.298**	-.184#	-.252***	-.279**	.059	-.227#
Region 7	-.066	-.203	-.272***	-.189	-.056	-.303**	-.185#	-.142	-.104	.172#	-.102
Region 8	-.090	-.165	-.163	.106	-.063	-.325*	-.121	-.308*	-.280**	-.112	-.152
Region 9	-.153	-.220#	-.255***	-.158	-.026	-.303**	.002	-.180#	-.119	.029	-.025
Region 10	-.034	-.154	-.055	.064	.024	-.181#	-.075	-.134	-.084	-.002	-.045
Public	.015	.025	.017	-.043	-.073	-.113	.087	-.061	-.013	-.114	-.053
Not for profit	-.096	-.030	.094	.142	.010	-.073	-.037	-.175***	-.123	-.063	-.063
Sole co-county provider	-.098	.076	.159	-.291**	.100	.020	-.022	.028	.008	.143#	.073
Number of beds	.068	-.087	.016	-.127	-.078	-.025	.174#	.001	.002	.032	.072
Starting salary	.048	-.034	-.168	.018	-.139	-.087	-.177#	-.126	-.163#	-.038	-.177
Percent salary increase	-.116	-.003	-.023	-.043	-.139	-.061	-.016	-.058	-.069	-.091	-.125
Relocation expense	.028	.176#	-.113	.068	-.015	.052	.037	-.055	-.043	.009	-.070
R-square adjusted	.020	0	.037	.063	0	.042	.078	.050	.034	0	0
F	1.2	0.8	1.3	1.5	0.7	1.4	1.8	1.5	1.3	1.0	0.8
Significance	NS	NS	NS	<.10	NS	NS	<.05	<.10	NS	NS	NS

NOTE: Data shown are standardized (beta) regression coefficients. Values for regions are relative to the omitted category, region 11. Values for ownership are relative to the omitted category, for profit.

*p < .001; **p < .01; ***p < .05; #p < .10.

would include expenditures for overtime, temporary staff, and recruitment of additional personnel. In addition to expenditures for the last mentioned of these, the survey also asked the hospitals their assessment of the competitiveness of their benefit package in the recruitment and retention process and the relative importance of various benefit options.

PROCEDURAL RESPONSES

A total of 42 (15%) responding hospitals indicated that they had closed some beds during calendar year 1988 in response to inadequate staffing. With regard to deviation from established standards, hospitals were asked for their assessment of the frequency of such deviations on a scale from 1 to 5, in which 1 would indicate that such deviation had not occurred at all and 5 would indicate that such deviation had occurred very frequently. Deviations from established standards with regard to the timing of admissions, transfers, surgery, and laboratory/X-ray procedures were reported as occurring sporadically, with mean scores in the range of 1.6 to 2.1. More widespread were deviations from established standards for the continuity of nurse assignments (mean score of 2.9), number of nursing hours per patient (3.0), and responsiveness to patient preferences (2.7).

FINANCIAL RESPONSES

Hospitals reported spending an average of nearly $300,000 on overtime, nearly $90,000 on recruiting, more than $730,000 on temporary staff from in-house agencies, and $568,000 on temporary staff from outside agencies during the year 1988. Because there was considerable variation in the number of hospitals reporting each type of expenditure, these figures cannot be aggregated into a comprehensive total—while a large majority reported expenditures on overtime (213) and recruitment (232), smaller numbers provided estimates of expenditures on temporary staff (68 for in-house, 188 for outside). Taking the expenditures for overtime and recruitment as being representative of the entire sample, and computing per hospital averages for temporary staff based on the number of hospitals indicating that they had used these services (121 in-house and 201 outside) and average expenditures for these categories, one would arrive at an average level of expenditures for personnel of nearly $1.1 million resulting directly or indirectly from the nurse shortage.[1]

RECRUITMENT AND RETENTION STRATEGIES

Ultimately, patient care of the highest quality is best ensured by the development and maintenance of a cadre of nursing personnel who are convinced that the hospital is dedicated to their well-being and is making every feasible effort to enhance their morale. This fact is hardly alien to the hospital industry in Florida, and the survey data provide information on those benefits that they consider to be most important in recruitment and retention, those benefit elements available that are deemed competitive in the marketplace, and those strategies that they actually employ to recruit and retain nursing personnel.

Five benefits—paid vacation, health insurance, sick pay, paid holidays, and a retirement program—are viewed (in that order) as being the most important elements in recruitment and retention. It is not surprising that these benefits represent five of the six elements (along with life insurance) that the responding hospitals felt were most competitive. At least three fourths of all hospitals felt that they were competitive with respect to these benefits. Other components of a benefits package that were considered competitive by a majority of hospitals included personal leave and tuition reimbursement (70%), paid Continuation Education Units (67%), and paid educational leave (53%). Also, not surprising, benefits such as paid sabbaticals, on-site housing, and day-care vouchers, which were considered as least important to recruitment and retention, were viewed as being competitive by less than 10% of the hospitals.

The actual responses of hospitals to the need to recruit and retain nursing personnel would include both enhancements to their own level of attractiveness to current and potential employees as well as efforts to attract the interest of nurses employed elsewhere or of persons about to embark on a career decision. Enhancements to attractiveness are grouped in Table 6.6 as being financial, educational, and other.

It is clear that hospitals are choosing to increase the level of salaries and to provide a broader range of salaries in order to deal with the issue of salary compression. Additionally, a wide variety of educational opportunities are afforded to upgrade and enhance the skills of nursing personnel. A great deal of flexibility of work hours

TABLE 6.6 Strategies of Enhancement Employed by Florida Hospitals

Financial		Educational		Other	
Strategy	Percentage Employing	Strategy	Percentage Employing	Strategy	Percentage Employing
Increased salary	98	Internships	56	Child care	47
Broadened salary		Preceptorships	75	Image enhancement	80
range	96	Tuition		In-house registry	66
Improved benefit		reimbursement	92	Weekend program	66
structure	76	In-service education	98	Part-time	93
On-site housing	16	Paid conference time	83	10- to 12-hour shifts	88
		Involvement in		4- to 6-hour shifts	51
		research	27	Counseling	47
		Computer training	44		

has become the norm, with greater part-time and weekend work as well as the possibility of working the regular number of hours per week in fewer days.

Hospitals also report many outreach programs, including direct mail (54%), newspaper (98%), and radio/TV (28%) advertising; job fairs (77%) and booths at conventions (66%); and special recruitment efforts directed at non-Florida and foreign nurses (71% and 43%, respectively). These could all be viewed as efforts to attract previously trained nurses into employment with the hospital. Another series of efforts are reported that are designed to attract newcomers into the nursing profession. These include career days (82%), career counseling services for secondary and college-age students (62%), open houses for students (61%), and programs about opportunities in nursing aimed at school guidance personnel (36%).

In the long run, it is precisely strategies such as these that will be necessary both to retain existing nursing personnel in their profession and to attract new entrants to nursing. For the individual hospital, it is difficult to argue that these strategies, if maintained for a considerable period of time, are not wholly appropriate. It is also important to realize, however, that there are real limitations on what any individual hospital can accomplish. Many of the strategies described here are designed to protect or increase the individual hospital's share of an existing labor force. Hospital-based programs aimed at acquainting students with the desirability of a

nursing career are faced with overcoming negative images and ste-
reotypes associated with nursing. Ultimately, the responsibility for
overcoming these images lies partially with the industry but especially with the profession itself (Schmeling, 1990).

Discussion

Findings from the survey of hospitals in Florida provide much
understanding of the shortage of nursing personnel both within the
state and nationally. One contributor to the shortage is the continuing increase in the demand for nurses, which exceeds any increase
in supply. Florida is a growing state, and the registered nurse population has continued to increase as well. The health care industry,
and especially hospitals, however, have contributed to increased
demand for nurses. Our findings demonstrate that nurse to patient
ratios increased from 1984 to 1987, when the shortage of personnel
reached a peak. To meet the demand for personnel and to compensate for vacancy and turnover in nursing staff, hospitals spent considerable amounts on overtime and on temporary staff from both
internal staffing pools and from freestanding staffing agencies. Although not a topic of this study, the recruitment of foreign nurses
continued; the Florida Hospital Association (1990) reported that
23% of its members seek nurses from abroad. Relatively few hospitals (15%) dealt with shortages in staff by closing beds or curtailing
services. Because empty beds are costly to the hospital, given their
fixed operating costs, resorting to this strategy as a means of coping
with shortage is less likely now than in earlier years, given the current business atmosphere of the hospital industry. Hospitals coped
with the staffing shortage by seeking other sources of personnel,
yet another indication that nursing demand had continued to grow.

The trend toward using in-house pools of staff is a reasonable
one in times of the need for efficiency in the use of personnel
(Bracken, Clakin, Sanders, & Thesen, 1985). Such resources enable
flexible staffing patterns and work hours for regular staff and per-
mit adjustments in labor costs to meet actual work load requirements that occur with fluctuations in occupancy. When Bracken et
al. (1985) evaluated hospital departments' work load with regard to
dependency on the patient census, nursing units were found to be
much more dependent than were units such as medical records and

accounting. In considering conditions for reducing operating expenses, nurse labor costs therefore become a highly flexible item. Particularly in areas of high tourism and seasonal population shifts affecting patient censuses, mechanisms for flexible staffing will appear much as those found in this study.

Another interesting feature of the nursing shortage was its uneven distribution throughout the geographic area of the study universe. The supply of nurses was not evenly distributed, nor was it congruent with current demand. Smaller institutions suffered disproportionately greater shortages than did medium-sized or large hospitals. This can be partially explained by lower salary levels in the rural areas, where many smaller hospitals are located. Larger facilities also have more flexibility for shifting assignments for the nurse who is dissatisfied, thereby deterring turnover as well.

Salaries were highly differentiated by geographic area. It was clear that salary levels followed local wage and cost-of-living levels, with highly urbanized areas paying higher salaries. Hospitals showed little recognition in salary levels for the basic educational preparation for the registered nurse. Because graduates of all three basic education programs generally available take the same examination, are licensed with the same credential, and function in similar assignments, salary differentiation for basic nursing education has not occurred. The small salary differences for nurses of differing basic educational preparation found here was consistent with the national averages found in 1988, which were $22,201 for associate degree graduates, $22,383 for diploma graduates, and $23,161 for baccalaureate graduates (*Seventh Report to the President and Congress*, 1990).

It is well documented that job dissatisfaction leads to the intent to leave, resulting in turnover and vacancy (Curry, Wakefield, Price, Mueller, & McCloskey, 1985; McCloskey, 1990; Prescott & Bowen, 1987). Prescott and Bowen learned that work load was an important determinant in the decision to resign. McCloskey and Curry et al. demonstrated the effect of autonomy in the workplace along with level of pay and work load. Our findings show that high turnover rates exist in an environment of decreased nurse-patient ratios in the last 12 months, relatively low wages, and disrupted continuity in the workplace due to the heavy use of part-time and temporary staff. On the other hand, the need to provide skills for more autonomy in the rapidly changing hospital environment is evident in the relatively generous educationally focused benefit packages offered by many hospitals. Hospitals are clearly sensitive to changes needed in the workplace to compete successfully for professional nurses at a time when the demand for them is steadily increasing.

Note

1. Some 121 hospitals reported the use of temporary staff from in-house agencies during 1988. If one assumes that the average expenditures of $730,281 for the 68 of these who were able to provide estimates of annual expenditures for this category are representative of all 121, then total annual expenditures would be $88.4 million, or $307,900 for each of the 287 hospitals in the survey. Similarly, some 201 hospitals reported the use of temporary staff from outside agencies during 1988. If one assumes that the average expenditures of $568,128 for the 188 of these who were able to provide estimates of annual expenditures for this category are representative of all 201, then total annual expenditures would be $114.2 million, or $397,900 for each of the 287 hospitals in the survey.

SEVEN

Nurses' Work in Nursing Homes

MARIE E. COWART

Nursing homes employed about 8% of active registered nurses in 1984 and 23% of licensed practical nurses in 1983 (National Institute on Aging, 1987, p. 56-A). This declined to 6% of employed registered nurses in 1988 (U.S. Department of Labor, 1990). Ancillary personnel are the predominant nursing personnel in nursing homes, constituting approximately 71% of the nursing staff, according to the 1985 National Nursing Home Survey (*Seventh Report to the President and Congress*, 1990). According to a similar study by the National Center for Health Statistics, licensed practical nurses made up 17% of the nursing staff in the nursing home, and registered nurses, 12%.

The nursing home setting holds dilemmas for the nurse seeking employment; among them are a changing client mix, low proportions of professional workers, documentation requirements, and low physician support coupled with the opportunities of an emerging professional specialty with the growing research literature about the care of the debilitated, long-term care client. The nursing home is one of the most heavily regulated of the health and social sector industries. Restrictive reimbursement through Medicaid, coupled with unaffordably high charges for private-pay residents, have contributed to the high regulatory environment that focuses largely on quality of care issues. For the most part, the nursing home care model follows a medical care model resulting in traditions in practice and client mix often not suited to the residential setting. These circumstances make the nursing home a challenging, yet exciting, place to work. Future prospects of increasing numbers of elderly and disabled predict an increasingly important role for the nursing home in the years to come.

In Florida, there are more than 500 nursing homes. We mailed questionnaires to the 474 nursing homes under the regulatory jurisdiction of the Florida Health Care Cost Containment Board and received responses from 460 for a 97.6% corrected response rate. The 52 homes affiliated with continuing care retirement communities (CCRCs) were not included; neither were 3 nursing homes associated with Veterans Administration hospitals. Nonresponses included one closed nursing home, two from undelivered mail, and twelve questionnaires not returned. Thus our sample is almost consistent with the population of nursing homes in the state with the exception of federal homes and those with CCRC affiliations. Such a sample reflects all of the diversity of the nursing home industry with homes of various sizes, ownership, and specialty interests. Of the 459 nursing homes in the sample reporting their number of beds, some 42 had fewer than 60 beds (9%), while 96 (21%) had at least 150 beds; 2 had in excess of 400 beds. The median size of the nursing homes was 128 beds, while the most frequent size was 120 beds. Nearly 90% were proprietary or under for-profit ownership. The geographic distribution of the nursing homes was generally similar to that of the population with some overrepresentation in the west coast St. Petersburg area and some underrepresentation of facilities in the Fort Lauderdale and Miami areas on the southeast coast. Eighteen (4.4%) were sole county providers of service, which means over one quarter of Florida's 67 counties were served with one nursing home. These were most frequently located in the rural areas in the central and northern parts of the state.

Nursing Staff Characteristics

The most notable feature of the nurses in nursing homes was their age. Older than the overall 39-year average age of employed nurses (*Seventh Report to the President and Congress*, 1990), nurses who worked in nursing homes were age 47.7 years on average. Less than 1% were under 25 years of age, but 9% were 65 years and over. In the smaller (0 to 59 beds) homes, there were more over-65-year-old nurses, and no nurses under the age of 25 years reported. Consistent with the older nurse, diploma education was most frequently reported (44%), with associate degree (33%) and baccalaureate degree preparation (20%) following; 3% of nurses working in nursing homes held a graduate degree. The high proportion of associate degree preparation is consistent with the strong community college system of nursing education programs enrolling older students in the state.

Staff Shortage

EXTENT OF THE SHORTAGE

In nursing homes, we examined the extent of the shortage using three measures: the perception of the nursing home administrator as to the seriousness of the shortage, the nurse-patient ratios, and the vacancy rates of the nursing staff.

Nursing home administrators were asked to assess the nurse staffing shortage on a scale of 1 to 5 in ascending order of perceived seriousness for a number of variables. The most serious shortages were reported for summer and winter months, weekends, and evening and night shifts. The summer shortages may be attributed to staff vacation leave, while winter shortages were most likely due to the increased bed occupancy documented by the Florida Health Care Cost Containment Board (1988b). The nursing assistant category was viewed as most severe in terms of availability. Table 7.1 reports findings on nursing home administrators' perceptions of the nursing shortage.

We found little difference in nurse-resident staffing ratios from 1984 to 1988, a period of slight surplus of nursing staff to a period of shortage beginning in 1987. However small, there was a steady decline in staff-resident ratios for both registered nurses and nursing assistants. The decline in the licensed practical nurse-resident ratios did not emerge until 1988, although this may have been due to downward substitution of the LPN for the registered nurse. These changes in staffing ratios were small, a factor thought to be due to the staffing standards required by the certification and licensure process. Despite the decline in nursing staffing ratios, it was during this period of the mid-1980s that the length of stay of residents in nursing homes shortened and acuity levels increased.

Nursing home vacancy rates were a reflection of the number of unfilled budgeted positions compared with the total number of budgeted positions available. Because vacancy rates were based on budget priorities, they reflected administrative planning and priorities rather than personnel availability. Due to regulatory staffing requirements, the vacancy rates for nursing staff for nursing homes

TABLE 7.1 Report of Ratings of Seriousness of the Nursing Shortage
According to Specific Characteristics in Florida Nursing
Homes, 1988

Characteristic	Industry Rating of Seriousness
Classification:	
RN	2.9
LPN	2.9
NA	3.1
Season:	
spring	3.0
summer	3.1
fall	3.0
winter	3.1
Day of the week:	
Wednesday	2.3
Saturday	3.8
Sunday	3.7
Shift:	
day	2.5
evening	3.5
night	3.3

NOTE: Seriousness scale: 1 = not serious and 5 = very serious.

were lower than those in other industries, particularly for the LPN
and nursing assistant (18% and 12%, respectively). On the other
hand, the RN vacancy rate was higher, at 25%, supporting the hypothesis of downward substitution of LPN personnel for RN staff.
Publicly owned nursing homes and the ones with the most beds
had the lowest vacancy rates. Homes with fewer than 60 beds had
the highest vacancy rates for all categories of nursing staff, although the smaller numbers of positions for nurses in these facilities create a greater impact with each position vacated.

Clearly, staffing ratio and vacancy data support the perceptions
of nursing home administrators regarding the shortage of nursing
personnel. Further examination of the data on causes of the shortage more dramatically describe the situation.

When data for vacancy rates was examined geographically by regression, nursing assistant rates were significant ($p = .10$), with the
highest rates in the St. Petersburg, Orlando, Fort Myers, and Miami

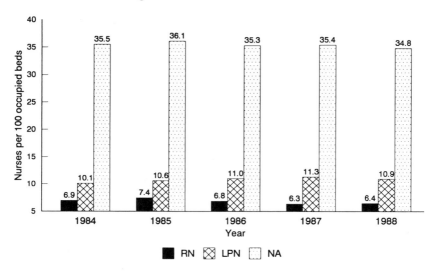

Figure 7.1. FTE Nursing Staff per 100 Occupied Beds in Florida Nursing Homes: 1984 to 1988

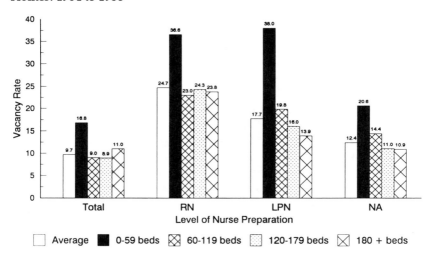

Figure 7.2. Vacancy Rates for Nursing Staff by Level of Preparation and Size of Nursing Home, Florida, 1988

areas. Smaller facilities had higher rates for the nursing assistant (p = .05, .001) and licensed practical nurse groups.

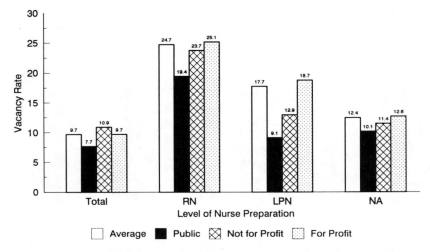

Figure 7.3. Vacancy Rates for Nursing Staff by Level of Preparation and Ownership in Florida Nursing Homes: 1988

CAUSES OF THE SHORTAGE

In this study, causes of the nursing shortage were examined using the variables of nursing staff turnover rates, beginning hourly salary levels, annual increases in salary, and percentage of the salary represented by the fringe benefit package. Compared with vacancy rates, turnover rates are a more accurate indicator of personnel satisfaction. We defined *turnover* as the number of full- and part-time staff who left employment in relation to the total number of budgeted positions for the nursing staff. All positions of the nursing staff were vacated at exceedingly high rates. Registered nurse positions turned over every 15 months on average (74.1 turnover rate) and licensed practical nurse positions vacated on average every 16 months (69.1 turnover rate). Most of the care of nursing home residents is carried out by the nursing assistant, however. Yet the turnover rates for this level of employee were 113.5 on average, or more than once yearly for every nursing assistant position in the nursing home. These alarming rates were even higher for the 40% of nursing homes with 120 to 179 beds, where the average turnover rate for nursing home assistants was 122.5, or about every 10 months. Clearly, such rates are indicative of

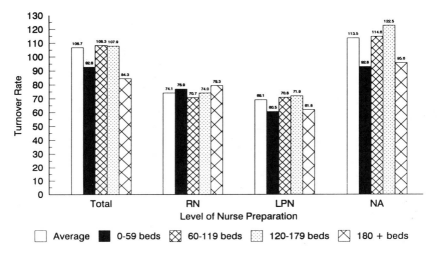

Figure 7.4. Turnover Rates for Nursing Staff by Level of Preparation and Size of Nursing Home, Florida, 1988

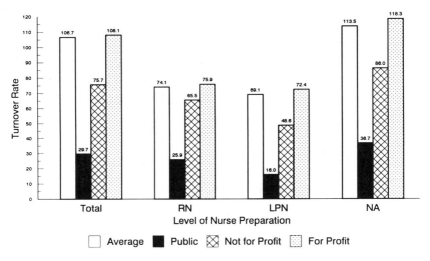

Figure 7.5. Turnover Rates for Nursing Staff by Level of Preparation and Ownership of Florida Nursing Homes: 1988

competition in the workplace and of job dissatisfaction of enormous proportions (Figures 7.4 and 7.5).

TABLE 7.2 Average Beginning Hourly Salary Levels for Nursing Staff
in Florida Nursing Homes According to DHRS District, 1988

| DHRS District | Average Hourly Salary Level (in dollars) RN Educational Preparation | | | | |
	A.D.N. Degree (n = 386)	Diploma (n = 367)	B.S.N. Degree (n = 319)	LPN (n = 440)	CNA (n = 444)
Average	9.96	9.95	10.11	8.63	5.04
1 (Pensacola)	9.57	9.00	9.07	7.17	4.28
2 (Tallahassee)	10.76	10.42	10.58	8.28	4.24
3 (Gainesville)	10.45	9.54	9.80	7.98	4.71
4 (Jacksonville)	10.48	9.80	9.99	8.33	4.75
5 (St. Petersburg)	10.31	9.53	9.69	8.81	5.31
6 (Tampa)	10.83	9.52	9.50	8.23	4.74
7 (Orlando)	10.71	9.46	9.74	8.38	5.04
8 (Fort Myers)	11.85	9.62	9.52	8.28	5.37
9 (West Palm Beach)	11.73	10.78	10.94	10.16	5.72
10 (Fort Lauderdale)	11.77	10.59	11.03	9.12	5.07
11 (Miami)	12.11	11.38	11.68	9.03	5.27

Like vacancy rates, when turnover rates were analyzed by analysis
of variance with regard to geographic location, the St. Petersburg,
West Palm Beach, Fort Lauderdale, and Miami areas were significant
($p = .05$). Regression analysis of turnover in relation to ownership of
the nursing home revealed significant findings for the LPN and nursing assistant in that turnover was lower in the not-for-profit homes.

Salaries and benefits were another area of inquiry. Salaries for the
registered nurse reflected little difference attributed to educational
preparation. Average starting salaries for the newly trained associate
degree-prepared registered nurse were $9.96 an hour in December 1988.
Nurses with diploma education began on average at $9.96 hourly, and
baccalaureate nurses, at $10.11. Licensed practical nurses were paid an
average of $8.63 hourly, and the nursing assistant, $5.04 (Table 7.2).

Closer examination showed differences in salaries according to
the size of the home. Larger homes reported more salaries for all
types of nursing personnel in the higher ranges than the smallest,
under-60-bed facilities. The latter reported more salaries for all categories of nursing personnel in lower hourly salary ranges.

Salaries for all levels of personnel follow local geographic area cost
of living and wages for other personnel. Salaries in the lower coastal

TABLE 7.3 Percentage of Annual Increase in the Starting Salaries of RNs According to Ownership of Florida Nursing Homes, 1988 (*n* = 330)

Percentage Starting Salary Increase	Percentage with Increase in Starting Salary for RNs Nursing Home Ownership		
	Public	Not for Profit	For Profit
15 or more	12.5	4.0	13.0
13-14	0.0	2.0	2.5
11-12	0.0	32.7	9.7
9-10	0.0	10.2	7.2
7-8	25.0	6.1	5.1
5-6	25.0	10.2	11.2
3-4	12.5	2.0	4.1
1-2	25.0	32.6	46.9
Average	6.0	8.0	5.0

portions of the state—West Palm Beach, Fort Lauderdale, and Miami—were higher than in the northern and western panhandle regions. When salaries are examined by the educational preparation of the nurse, nurses with baccalaureate preparation made 15 cents more hourly than diploma or associate degree nurses. By ownership, by far the largest proportion of nursing homes are proprietary, many associated with national firms. Salaries for nurses employed in the for-profit facilities were lower than in the public or not-for-profit homes. Turnover for the for-profit firms was also higher for all categories of nursing personnel.

During the same period, the median rate of increase in the starting salary for registered nurses who were employed by nursing homes was 5.1%, nearly two full percentage points above that for nursing assistants. For RNs employed in not-for-profit nursing homes, the average increase in starting salary was 8%, clearly above the raise for RNs in either public or proprietary facilities (Table 7.3). For both LPNs and nursing assistants, the median increase in starting salaries in the for-profit sector, at 5% and 4%, respectively, was less than in homes with other types of ownerships.

In terms of fringe benefit packages, there were alarming findings related to inability to attract personnel to nursing homes. Fringe benefit packages ranged from 1% to 30% of the salary; the mean was 15.9% for registered nurses, 16.2% for licensed practical nurses, and 16.8% for the nursing assistant. Modal benefits were between 12% and 15% of the salary for all categories of personnel. For the LPN, benefits were significantly higher in the St. Petersburg, Sarasota, West Palm Beach, and Fort Lauderdale areas when examined by analysis of variance (significance = .10). Less than 30% of nursing home administrators indicated retirement benefits were important to recruitment of personnel; and, when interviewed, select staff nurses in nursing homes indicated they were just beginning to plan for providing pension benefits in their homes (Speake, Cowart, & Schmeling, 1990b). Nursing home administrators ranked retirement packages behind benefits for vacation, health insurance, sick pay, and holidays when asked their opinion about the importance of retirement benefits. The value of the benefits package was inversely related to turnover for the registered nurse when regression analysis was conducted (p = .001).

High turnover rates clearly related to the nursing shortage result in interruptions of productivity during recruitment and orientation. Such slowdowns in productivity place greater burdens for resident care on the remaining staff, contributing to their dissatisfaction and creating a cycle of turnover and shortage. Low salaries and minimal annual salary increases provide little incentive for attracting or retaining staff. Small fringe benefit packages, often without pension or retirement benefits, provide few supplements to the unattractive salaries and further contribute to the difficulty in attracting and retaining personnel.

IMPACTS OF THE NURSING SHORTAGE

Despite shortages of staff, vacancy rates in nursing homes were maintained at moderate to low levels; in 1988, only 2 of 460 reporting homes were forced to temporarily close beds. To explore further, however, nursing home administrators were asked whether other established standards of practice were altered because of staff shortages. They indicated that standards for continuity of assignments, patient satisfaction, responsiveness to patient preferences, and number of nursing hours per patient were deviated from on a frequent basis. They also indicated that rates of falls, infections, medication errors, transfers, and admissions were affected.

Nursing homes also spent an average of $55,400 on overtime expense. Almost half, or $25,605, was spent on nursing assistants, a further indication of the seriousness of the shortage for this category of personnel. Use of overtime according to the amount of over-

TABLE 7.4 Strategies for Enhancing Recruitment and Retention of Nursing Personnel Used by Nursing Home Administrators

Financial Strategy	*Percentage Employing*	*Educational* Strategy	*Percentage Employing*	*Other* Strategy	*Percentage Employing*
Increased salary	97	Internships	18	Child care	16
Broadened salary		Preceptorships	19	Image enhancement	54
range	85	In-service education	88	In-house registry	26
		Paid conference time	69	Weekend program	38
		Involvement in research	7	Part-time	79
		Computer training	11	10- to 12-hour shifts	44
				4- to 6-hour shifts	33
				Counseling	26

time expense reported was also significantly affected by the geographic location of the nursing home. Such expenses were generally at their highest in the central and southeastern portions of the state.

In addition to overtime expense, nursing homes reported they spent on average $11,216 for recruitment expense with the director of nursing assuming the role of recruiter (Speake, Cowart, & Schmeling, 1990b).

STRATEGIES

Correction of the high turnover rates among all levels of nursing personnel in nursing homes can be accomplished in part through offering attractive benefits packages during the recruitment process as well as to existing personnel. Administrators were asked to rate various benefits in terms of their value in recruiting and retaining personnel. Homes used increased salary, wider salary ranges, and in-service education for recruitment (Table 7.4).

Discussion

The nursing home provides a unique employment setting for the registered nurse. Clearly, the older nurse is attracted to this setting. Whether the individual is one recently prepared in an associate degree program or is midway in the career and chooses to work in the nursing home setting is an area for further exploration. We suspect that both situations occur. High turnover rates, however, indicate that the conditions of work are not as expected or other forms of dissatisfaction occur to cause the nurse to leave the setting. Seven-day, 24-hour staff coverage for care is not easily provided even in times when there are adequate personnel. In times of personnel shortages, coverage for weekends, evenings, and nights becomes an acute burden on permanent staff. Seasonal shifts in census have become more evident in nursing homes with shorter lengths of stay and emphasis on rehabilitative care rather than residential care; thus winter months are difficult to staff. Summer staffing difficulties may be due to vacation leave and absence of part-time workers.

Evidence of the regulation of the nursing home appeared in the nurse-resident staffing ratios. It may also have affected some findings. Questionnaires were sent to nursing homes in Florida under the regulatory authority of the Florida Health Care Cost Containment Board. Because the responses to the questionnaires became public information, we learned through anecdotes that nursing home administrators were reluctant to report some of the impacts of the nursing home shortage such as higher staffing ratios and errors in care. During the 1984 to 1988 period, some substitution of LPN for RN staff was found. While our study did not provide strong evidence of the impact of the nursing shortage and vacancies on quality of care, Munroe (1990) found that nursing homes with a higher ratio of RN hours to LPN hours per resident day demonstrated modestly higher levels of quality of care. Thus some of the means of coping with the shortage were felt to be underreported.

Moderate vacancy rates contrasted markedly with the high turnover rates. On first glance, if vacancy rates alone were used as an indicator of shortage, minimal problems in staffing could be inferred. Again, however, the regulatory policy for minimal staffing provides a stimulus unique to this health industry to fill positions as they become vacant. Turnover tells the truer story of continual churning of the pool of nursing staff for the home.

In our study, all categories of nurses had high turnover rates. Stryker (1982) examined turnover of nursing personnel in 37 nursing homes in the St. Paul and Minneapolis areas during a two-year period. When queried, nursing staff indicated reasons for leaving were job competition (28%), personal reasons (24%), discharged (20%), the job itself (17%), and returned to school (11%). More than half of the participating homes were successful in reducing turn-over by implementing management techniques of improved supervision of new employees, supervisory training, revised personnel policies, increased recruitment efforts, and avoidance of use of personnel pools.

Turnover is a costly activity causing added expense for recruitment, hiring, orientation, extra supervision, and development to full productivity of the new worker. Wise (1990) estimates the cost of the turnover of one registered nurse in the hospital setting to be $13,000, with the estimated time of development to full productivity from 3 to 18 months. Documentation of the cost of turnover for all levels of nursing home personnel is needed.

Nursing assistants provide the majority of the care of the resident of the nursing home. This low-wage worker is usually female and often minority. McCulloch (1989) found that 5% of 1,500 nursing assistants in Florida responding to her survey were male, and 55% were black. The average age of the nursing assistants she interviewed was 38 years, and half were single heads of households, with one third of all respondents single parents caring for a total of more than 1,000 children under 16 years of age. Her findings on salary and fringe benefits are consistent with ours. Some three quarters of the nursing assistant respondents earned between $4.00 and $6.00 hourly, and almost two thirds had no retirement benefits. Some were part-time workers. The usual work load for the nursing assistant ranges from 9 to 12 residents daily, providing their full hygienic and mobility care for the day. For the registered nurse and licensed practical nurse, competing employers are the hospital and other health care employers. For the nursing assistant, the competing employers are more likely to be the hospitality industries. Comparisons of the work load and status of the employee in the nursing home with those of hotel or restaurant employment can shed some light on the extremely high turnover rates for this category of personnel. Adding to the heavy work load and responsibility of care are new requirements for certification, modest salaries with low salary raises, and minimal benefits often excluding retirement programs.

Waxman, Carner, and Berkenstock (1984) found contrasting findings when high annual turnover rate for nursing assistant staff were found in higher quality homes. At the same time, aides from these same homes reported the highest job satisfaction scores. The authors indicate that further analysis led to one explanation: Where aides perceived the nursing home environment as highly ordered, organized and structured turnover rates were higher than in homes wherein the aides perceived the administration as being more flexible and loosely organized. Thus management style was proported as more directly influencing turnover than other variables. More recently, Grau, Chandler, Burton, and Kilditz (1991) found that the quality of the social environment of the nursing home was as important as attitudes toward job benefits in accounting for institutional loyalty among nursing assistants.

Salaries in nursing homes were low, with an average of $9.54 per hour for the beginning registered nurse. This compares with a median salary of approximately $21,300 in 1987 for the registered nurse in the nursing home, according to a survey by the Hospital Compensation Service, Hawthorne, New Jersey (U.S. Department of Labor, 1990). The Hospital Compensation Service also reported that licensed practical nurses in nursing homes earned a median annual salary of $15,000 in 1987; certified nursing aides, $16,600; and noncertified nursing aides, about $10,400 in 1988. The 1989 average nursing home hourly wage, according to the American Health Care Association, was $12.26 for registered nurses, $9.18 for licensed practical nurses, and $4.85 for nursing assistants—appreciably higher than our 1988 data indicating low salary levels for nursing home nursing staff in Florida (reported by Mohler & Lessard, 1990).

Theisen and Pelfrey (1990) found that employee benefit plans can be used for recruiting and retaining nurses. Because most nursing home personnel work for fewer fringe benefits than nurses in other settings (Serow & Cowart, 1990), enhancement of the benefits package, particularly pension benefits, could positively affect retention of staff. Tax deferral methods of providing retirement plans can be implemented at little cost to the nursing home's operations (Theisen & Pelfrey, 1990), although plans having employer contributions are of greater benefit to the employee, particularly the low-wage nursing assistant who probably can little afford wage deferment plans. Career advancement mechanisms such as career ladders for nursing assistants have been used effectively in retaining nursing assistants (Rajecki, 1990) and are a cost effective method for improving staff continuity.

Findings about the importance of the workplace environment are beginning to appear in the literature. McCloskey (1990) found that nurses with low autonomy and low social integration reported low job satisfaction and work motivation, poor commitment to the organization, and less intent to stay on the job. The literature (Grau et al., 1991; McCloskey, 1990; McCulloch, 1989; Speake, Cowart, & Schemling, 1990b; Waxman et al., 1984) seems to confirm that management style, opportunities for autonomy, and a feeling of community are essential for retention of personnel in the nursing home setting. Hay's (1977) study of 100 superior nursing homes indicated that the nursing home administrator played a key role in establishing the overall "climate" of care in the nursing home. Thus training for nursing home administrators needs to incorporate human resource management skills as part of a comprehensive program to improve retention of nursing personnel.

Clearly, the demand for nursing home personnel will continue to grow. Corrections in personnel policies and management are needed as a first step to assure that nursing homes will capture an ample share of the available nursing personnel.

EIGHT

Community Employment Settings

MARIE E. COWART

DIANNE L. SPEAKE

Over time, the proportion of nurses employed in the community has increased. Once the major employment opportunities for nurses were the hospital and private duty nursing; now the proliferation of community service agencies has expanded employment opportunities for nurses outside the hospital setting. From 1984 to 1988, the number of registered nurses employed by non-hospital-based home health agencies increased 17% according to the *Seventh Annual Report to the President and Congress on the Status of Health Personnel in the United States* (1990). The number of ambulatory care settings expanded from 1984 to 1988 and, during this period, the number of registered nurses employed in those settings increased by 29%. Such settings included group practice physician offices, freestanding clinics, ambulatory surgical centers, and health maintenance organizations. Despite marked increases in these settings, little change occurred in nurse employment in the public health setting from 1984 to 1988. As hospitals experience the need to limit the number of beds designated for inpatient services, the number of employment opportunities for nurses outside the inpatient, acute care setting are likely to continue to increase.

In this chapter, we share findings about nurse employment in three important community settings: the certified home health care agency, the traditional public health agency, and the hospice. The findings concern trends in use of the nurse in these settings, information about nursing assistants, vacancy and turnover rates, salary and benefit information, and other related data. Comparisons of similarities and differences in employment in the three settings are discussed.

Home Health Agencies

From 1978 to 1988, the number of home health agencies doubled. Such settings provide increased options for nurse employment as well as increased opportunities for autonomy in practice and desirable work hours because evening and weekend hours are scheduled only occasionally or on an "on-call" basis. Such employment options are expected to expand in the future as trends for "aging in place" and community-based care increase. It is important to examine the employment practices of nurses in this evolving and expanding setting because it can be presumed that the home health agency directly competes for nurses with hospitals and other health care services.

In Florida, there are about 554 home health agencies. Questionnaires were sent to the agencies: 46 questionnaires were undelivered, 18 agencies had closed, and 42 agencies did not meet the predetermined criterion of providing "intermittent home visits." In addition, 7 were new facilities opened during the last quarter of 1988 or early 1989 and could not provide requested data. Responses were received from 416 (75%). Of these, many provided incomplete questionnaires. It was determined that 212 questionnaires were complete enough to be included in the study (48% corrected response rate).

Of the 191 home health agencies reporting, the average daily census was 85.5 clients (range of 1 to 1,073) during the week of December 5-11, 1988. The average number of home visits for the 1988 calendar year was 23,447. Most of the agencies studied were under for-profit ownership (63%) while 33% were not for profit and 4% were publicly owned. Nineteen agencies (or 9%) reported they were hospital based. The geographic location of home health agencies was similar to that of the population distribution in Florida. Only four agencies indicated that they were sole county providers of services. In addition to intermittent home visits, all agencies reported they provided at least one additional service; among them were private duty home health care, registry services, and temporary staffing services. In comparing the sample with the nonusable responses, there is some underrepresentation of small agencies. County public health units had over 2 million patient contacts in 1988, including 117,000 home visits. Ten county health units were certified home health agencies and were included in the study of home health agencies.

TABLE 8.1 Nursing Staff FTE Ratio to Average Daily Census in Florida Home Health Agencies, 1984 to 1988

Nursing Staff	1984	1985	1986	1987	1988
Total	0.34	0.46	0.53	0.45	0.46
	(n = 37)	(n = 62)	(n = 86)	(n = 131)	(n = 160)
RN	0.18	0.34	0.30	0.26	0.24
	(n = 38)	(n = 64)	(n = 91)	(n = 137)	(n = 196)
LPN	0.06	0.18	0.21	0.29	0.40
	(n = 20)	(n = 19)	(n = 36)	(n = 58)	(n = 141)
HHA	0.14	0.39	0.57	0.32	0.37
	(n = 34)	(n = 58)	(n = 77)	(n = 113)	(n = 75)

More of the nursing staff of the home health agencies were prepared in associate degree nursing education programs rather than diploma or baccalaureate settings. About a third of the nurses were under 35 years of age, and about 10% were over 55 years old. The median age was 39.9 years.

The nursing staff had a relatively short tenure of employment, with 88.4% reporting less than five years employment with their current agency and only 3% employed with the same agency for more than ten years. Considering the recent proliferation of newly opened home health firms, this finding was not surprising. Nurse staffing ratios indicated that overall staffing in relation to daily census increased slightly from .34 to .46 FTE total nursing staff per client from 1984 to 1988 (Table 8.1). Further statistical analysis by regression demonstrated that the size of nursing staff was larger in the agencies affiliated with a national chain. Further exploration of staffing ratios for the registered nurse, licensed practical nurse, and home health aide, however, showed greater increases in the use of the licensed practical nurse during the four-year period than in use of the registered nurse. The 1986 staffing ratios were greater for the RN and home health aide than those for other years. The decline of the registered nurse to daily census ratio from 1986 to 1988 and the increased use of the licensed practical nurse in the same period are indicators of the staffing shortage in the responding home health agencies.

Administrators reported more serious shortages of nursing personnel for registered nurses than for the licensed practical nurse or home health aide. It is not surprising that they ranked shortages more serious in winter months and for weekend, evening, and night shifts.

TABLE 8.2 Vacancy Rates for Nursing Staff by Size of Agency in
Florida Home Health Agencies, 1988

Nursing Staff	n	Average	0-49	Size of Agency by Daily Census 50-99	100-149	150+
Total	69	24.5	29.1	22.5	25.3	18.4
RN	80	31.2	39.8	27.1	27.5	24.1
LPN	110	83.3	88.8	84.0	88.7	69.5
HHA	19	44.5	58.5	36.4	75.0*	24.3

*One response.

Further evidence of the shortage of nurses was provided in the
vacancy and turnover rates of the nursing staff (Tables 8.2 to 8.5).
Vacancy rates were measured by the number of full- and part-time
unfilled budgeted positions in relation to the total number of budgeted positions. Turnover rates were represented by the number of
full- and part-time staff who left employment in relation to the total
number of budgeted positions. Reported nurse vacancy rates indicated the number of budgeted staff positions that were vacant at
the end of 1988. The lowest reported vacancy rates were for the registered nurse, at 31.2%, while the home health aide positions were
44.5% vacant and the licensed practical nurse positions were 83.3%
vacant. Larger agencies had lower vacancy rates for all levels of
nursing personnel than smaller agencies. Rates by ownership
showed little difference, although hospital-based agencies had the
lowest and public agencies reported the highest vacancies for the
LPN and the RN. What remains unknown is whether the higher vacancy rates for licensed practical nurses are due to a shortage of

TABLE 8.3 Vacancy Rates for Nursing Staff by Ownership of Agency in
Florida Home Health Agencies, 1988

Nursing Staff	n	Average	Public	Ownership of Agency Not for Profit	For Profit
Total	73	26.7	24.1	24.7	21.3
RN	83	36.7	32.6	30.1	29.7
LPN	116	91.7	85.6	82.9	78.1
HHA	19	*	36.6	48.2	30.2

*No response.

TABLE 8.4 Turnover Rates for Nursing Staff by Size of Agency in Florida Home Health Agencies, 1988

| Nursing Staff | n | Average | Size of Agency by Daily Census | | | |
			0-49	50-99	100-149	150+
Total	119	42.6	54.6	40.0	34.2	34.2
RN	136	51.9	69.7	42.6	42.8	39.4
LPN	64	29.9	29.3	45.7	20.5	21.6
HHA	33	67.4	93.5	33.9	113.1	35.0

applicants or a reluctance by home health agency administrators to fill budgeted positions.

Turnover rates for nursing staff in home health agencies was relatively high, with an overall average of 42.6%. Yet, for the LPN, turnover rates were lower than average, at 29.9%, but much higher for the RN and home health aide, at 51.9% and 67.4%. Again, smaller home health agencies had higher turnover than larger agencies, and for-profit agencies had higher rates than not-for-profit and publicly owned agencies. Thus, once filled, LPNs stayed in their positions longer than other nursing personnel.

Salaries and benefits were reported by the responding agencies. Starting hourly salaries for registered nurses with associate degree preparation were on average $11.31; for the licensed practical nurse, the starting salary was on average $9.18 an hour. These salaries were somewhat higher in the smaller agencies (0-49 census) at an average of $12.33 hourly compared with an average at larger agencies of $10.25 hourly. The same trend was evident in the salaries of licensed practical nurses in that the average in the smallest agencies was $9.56 hourly while, in the largest agencies, the average salary

TABLE 8.5 Turnover Rates for Nursing Staff by Ownership of Agency in Florida Home Health Agencies, 1988

| Nursing Staff | n | Average | Ownership of Agency | | |
			Public	Not for Profit	For Profit
Total	119	42.6	19.8	39.5	44.4
RN	136	51.9	39.0	48.7	54.8
LPN	64	29.9	7.6*	31.3	29.6
HHA	116	67.4	—	46.2	72.1

*One response.

was $8.05 hourly. For-profit agencies reported the highest average hourly salary levels for registered nurses, at $11.84, while not-for-profit agencies reported the lowest average hourly salaries, at $10.24. A similar trend was reported for the licensed practical nurse. Regression analysis demonstrated that public and for-profit starting salaries for the licensed practical nurse were significantly higher than those in the not-for-profit agencies.

Salaries varied by local geographic markets with the lowest salaries reported in the more rural northern part of the state and the highest salaries reported in the southern coastal portions of the state. The annual increase in starting salary for the nursing staff was 9.0% on average for the registered nurse and home health aide but an average of 11.4% for the licensed practical nurse. Publicly owned agencies trailed the not-for-profit and for-profit agencies with an average 3.0% annual salary increase. The smallest agencies reported the highest salary increases, about 1% higher than that for the agencies overall. Annual salary increases were by far higher for the northwest (Pensacola) and mid-Gulf coast (St. Petersburg) areas at an average of some 14% salary increase for the year.

The average value of the fringe benefit package for nursing staff employed in home health agencies was surprisingly high but varied among categories of nursing personnel. The percentage of salary represented in the fringe benefit package for the registered nurse was 20.6%; for the licensed practical nurse, 18.5%; and for the home health aide, 23.2%, on average. Ranges for all categories were from 0.0% to more than 36% of the value of the salary. With relatively high fringe benefit packages, only half of the responding agencies reported they provided retirement benefits for their employees.

Other data on the adequacy of the nursing personnel resources were collected. For example, home health agency administrators indicated that continuity of assignments and responsiveness to patient preferences were deviated from moderately because of the shortage of personnel. Less frequently, other areas of deviation from established practice due to the supply of nursing staff were the number of nursing hours per patient, patient satisfaction, and rate of medication errors and other reported incidents.

Home health agency administrators indicated they spent, on average, $21,360 in 1988 for overtime expense for nursing staff. The largest proportion went to the registered nurse, with home health aide overtime contributing the second highest expense item. Recruitment of

TABLE 8.6 Strategies for Enhancing Recruitment and Retention of Nursing Personnel Used by Home Health Agency Administrators

Financial		Educational		Other	
Strategy	*Percentage Employing*	*Strategy*	*Percentage Employing*	*Strategy*	*Percentage Employing*
Increased salary	91	Internships	29	Child care	33
Broadened salary range	84	Preceptorships	34	Image enhancement	70
		In-service education	84	In-house registry	—
		Paid conference time	74	Weekend program	—
		Involvement in research	16	Part-time	85
		Computer training	22	10- to 12-hour shifts	—
				4- to 6-hour shifts	—
				Counseling	32

personnel was also a required expense for the home health agency with an average of $16,779 reported for 1988 for 10 of the 212 reporting agencies; 133 agencies, however, indicated they spent an average of $7,500 annually in advertising for personnel. Less than a third of home health agencies reported they used temporary staff to supplement their regular nursing staff to provide services in the same year. About one fifth used in-house pool temporary staff, however, and about 15% used a freestanding temporary staffing agency for supplemental staff. Of those agencies using in-house pool staff, an average of $125,000 was spent; for those agencies using an outside agency, an average expense of $40,000 per agency was reported. Thus overtime and temporary staff expenses indicated inadequate regular staff to meet the demand for services for some agencies. Not clear from the data is whether these expenses are incurred because of the unavailability of applicants for vacant positions or because of temporary variances in patient caseload that do not indicate the need to hire permanent staff. The relatively low recruitment expense may indicate the latter is more likely for the home health agency.

As was the case for nursing homes (see Chapter Seven), it might be possible to lower the turnover rates among all levels of nursing personnel in home health agencies in part by offering desirable benefits packages during the recruitment process as well as to existing personnel (Table 8.6).

Public Health Nursing

Public health nursing services in Florida are provided by 67 county public health units (CPHUs) located in 11 health districts in the state. Personnel in the county health units are members of the state-wide career service system and are employees of the Florida Department of Health and Rehabilitative Services (DHRS). Local county health unit administrators and nursing directors have direct authority for hiring, promoting, and firing nurses in this system. Authority for county health unit services is jointly derived from state legislation and county ordinances, with funding supplied by federal, state, and county sources.

Questionnaires were not sent to individual county public health units, but aggregated data were obtained from computerized records of the Department of Health and Rehabilitative Services Personnel Office and the State Health Office. The registered nurses employed in county public health units were found to be better educated than nurses in hospitals, nursing homes, home health agencies, and hospitals, with twice the number (40%) of baccalaureate degrees and almost three times (8%) the number of graduate degrees than the other settings reported in this study. These figures are comparable to data indicating 37% of nurses employed in public health nationally have a baccalaureate degree (U.S. Department of Health and Human Services, 1990). This higher level of education is expected because public health nursing is generally offered only in baccalaureate and higher degree programs. In examining the state public health nurse classification system, a baccalaureate degree is usually required for community health nurses who provide school and field visits (home care) and for higher management and clinical positions. Registered nurses who function in a clinic setting, primarily in the Registered Nurse and Senior Registered Nurse classes, are not required to have baccalaureate degrees.

Tremendous growth in the number of health services provided by county public health units occurred during the 1980s. Figures 8.1 and 8.2 indicate a 38% growth in public health nursing visits between 1984 and 1989. In contrast, the growth in nurse FTEs was approximately half this amount.

Vacancy rates in county health units in 1988 were 20.5% for registered nurse budgeted positions, 11.1% for licensed practical nurses, and 11.9% for nursing assistants—levels lower than that found in

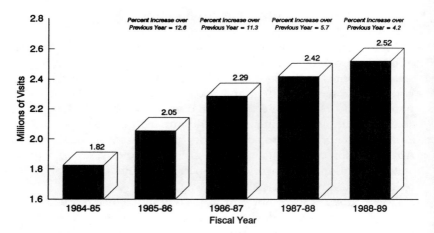

Figure 8.1. Public Health Nursing Visits by HRS County Public Health
Units: Fiscal Years 1984-1985 to 1988-1989
SOURCE: State Health Office, Florida Department of Health and Rehabilitative Services.

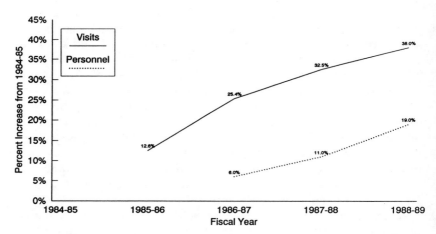

Figure 8.2. Cumulative Percentage of Increase in Public Health Nursing
Visits and Nurse Personnel (county public health units relative to 1984-1985)
SOURCE: State Health Office, Florida Department of Health and Rehabilitative Services.

Florida hospitals, nursing homes, and home health agencies. As salaries and benefits began to rise dramatically in the other settings

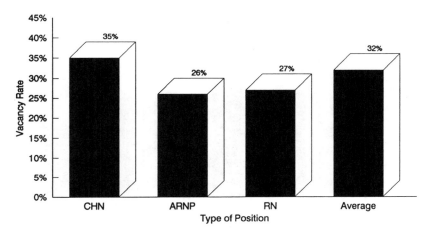

Figure 8.3. Vacancy Rates of Selected Nursing Positions for HRS County Public Health Units: June 30, 1990
SOURCE: State Health Office, Florida Department of Health and Rehabilitative Services.

during 1989 and 1990, however, the vacancy rates in CPHUs soared to 31.5% for the five public health direct service registered nurse classifications (Registered Nurse, Senior Registered Nurse, Community Health Nurse, Senior Community Health Nurse, and Advanced Registered Nurse Practitioner; see Figure 8.3).

The turnover rate in 1989 for the 2,046.5 registered nurses employed in public health nursing service classifications was 14.3% after adjusting for promotions, transfers, retirement, and death. The 1990 turnover rate for the same five classifications was 18.7% compared with only 9.8% for management and supervisory positions, indicating a greater tendency for nurses providing direct patient care to leave public health nursing positions.

Starting hourly salaries for registered nurses and licensed practical nurses in public health were as much as 25% lower than those for beginning nurses in home health agencies and they also trailed beginning salaries in the other settings—hospitals and nursing homes. The average beginning hourly rates were $8.32 for the RN and $7.15 for the LPN in 1988. The annual salary increase for that year was about 5% for all levels of state-employed nursing personnel in public health. Benefits were more competitive, at 22%, but

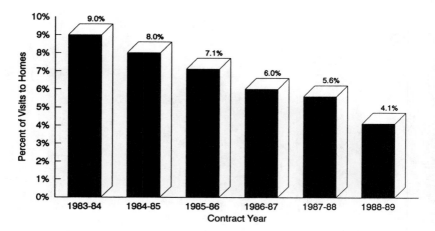

Figure 8.4. Home Visits as a Percentage of Total Visits by HRS County Public Health Units: Contract Years 1983-1984 to 1988-1989
SOURCE: State Health Office, Florida Department of Health and Rehabilitative Services.

the state retirement program was a strong component of the benefit program.

Several explanations for the rise in registered nurse vacancy and turnover rates are plausible. First, public health nurse salaries were at one time more competitive with other health care institutions in Florida. In 1988, however, public health registered nurse average beginning salaries trailed other settings by $1.64 to $2.99 per hour, or as much as 26%. The greatest difference in salaries was with home health agencies, a setting with greater similarity in nursing practice than hospitals or nursing homes. The fringe benefit package for registered nurses in county health units was competitive with home health agencies, with benefits valued at 22.0% of public health nurse salaries compared with a 20.6% value of home health agency registered nurse salaries. While the benefit packages for county public health unit licensed practical nurses exceeded home health agency benefits for LPNs, nursing assistants received less in benefits—20.0% compared with 23.2%, respectively.

Second, nurse salaries in public health agencies are directly linked to state career service salary structures and therefore are less responsive to market demands than those of the other health industries. Annual salary increases for registered nurses were higher in

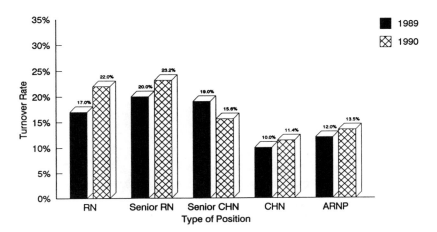

Figure 8.5. Turnover Rates of Selected Nursing Positions for Florida (Department of Health and Rehabilitative Services): December 1989 and 1990
SOURCE: State Health Office, Florida Department of Health and Rehabilitative Services.
NOTE: These turnover rates do not include separations due to retirement, death, dismissal, reassignment, transfer, promotion, or demotion.

hospitals (8.5%), nursing homes (5.1%), and home health agencies (9.0%) than were those for public health nurses (5.0%). The dramatic increase in vacancy rates in June 1990 followed the 1990 legislative session in which the legislature failed to remedy the widening gap in salaries between public health nurses and nurses in other health care settings.

A third explanation involves the changes occurring in public health nursing practice. Figure 8.4 indicates that the number of home visits by public health nurses has decreased dramatically between 1983 and 1989. More emphasis has been placed on clinic visits as the demand for public health services has grown. The introduction of primary, episodic health care for the indigent in county public health units has placed further demands on clinic services in county public health units. Nurses who once entered public health to provide health promotion and preventive services to a caseload of clients find that the milieu of public health nursing is changing. This observation is supported by Figure 8.5, which shows that the turnover rates for nurses employed primarily in clinics (RN, Senior RN) are higher than for those with greater practice autonomy and diversity

TABLE 8.7 Average Daily Census and Total Visits for Hospices, 1984 to 1988

Year	Number of Agencies	Average Daily Census	Annual Visits
1988	29	81.8	12,766
1987	25	50.9	7,311
1986	22	40.8	4,614
1985	18	26.4	2,571
1984	13	21.4	1,890

(CHNs, Senior CHNs, and ARNPs). Studies by Motaz (1988) further support the idea that job turnover is higher for employees who have less challenging job assignments, less autonomy, and fewer extrinsic rewards (salary and fringe benefits).

Finally, the introduction of evening and weekend primary health clinics and the on-call status of nurses working with substance-abused newborns and foster shelter children have eliminated another benefit of public health nursing—a Monday through Friday work schedule.

Hospices

The hospice industry is one that has emerged and expanded in the United States with the passage of federal legislation providing Medicare reimbursement for hospice services for the terminally ill. The total number of licensed hospices in Florida in 1988 was 32. On mailing questionnaires to these agencies, two were undelivered and we learned that one hospice had merged with a local home health agency and was reported as a part of the parent agency. Thus the 29 responses constituted a 100% corrected response rate.

For the 29 hospices reporting their daily censuses, the average was 81.8 clients with a range from 5 to 477 clients during the week of December 5-11, 1988. Almost half of the responding hospices indicated their average daily census fell between 50 and 99 patients. The average number of client visits for the 1988 calendar year was 12,766. The recent growth of this service was illustrated by the growth in average daily census and number of total visits per year from 1984 to 1988 (Table 8.7).

TABLE 8.8 Vacancy and Turnover Rates for Nurses Employed in Hospices, 1988

| | Vacancy Rates | | Turnover Rates | |
Nursing Staff	n	Average	n	Average
RN	29	7.20	23	28.34
LPN	11	9.35	6	54.62
NA	26	9.31	12	33.84

All 29 hospices indicated their ownership was private, not for profit; 4 were hospital based. None was affiliated with national firms; that is, all had been established locally. Eighteen (or 65.2%) were sole county providers of hospice services. The geographic distribution of the reporting hospices showed greater representation in the middle portion of the state and underrepresentation in the Miami area.

Hospices reported the educational backgrounds of nurses employed in their facilities: Half had associate degree preparation, one fourth had diploma nursing preparation, and one fourth a B.S.N. or graduate degree in nursing. The age distribution of nurses working in hospices showed a median age of 43.0 years with about one fifth under age 35 and about 15% over age 55 years. Most (92%) of the nursing staff of the hospices had been employed less than five years, while less than 4% were reported to have been employed for more than ten years.

Vacancy and turnover rates were examined as indicators of the extent of shortage and job dissatisfaction among nursing personnel (Table 8.8). Vacancy rates for all levels of nursing staff were relatively low, while turnover rates indicated that one third of RN and nursing assistant positions turned over each year. Such turnover occurred in half of LPN positions.

Salaries and benefits were reported for the nursing staff of the 29 hospices in 1988. The average starting salary for the associate degree-prepared registered nurse was $10.01 hourly in 1988. There were small differences observed in the starting salaries for nurses with diploma, baccalaureate, or graduate education: Starting hourly salaries for those nurses were $9.98, $9.99, and $9.88, on average, respectively. There was little difference between starting and maximum hourly salaries for the four educational levels of registered nurse.

The average maximum salary for the associate degree-prepared nurse was $12.48; for the diploma-prepared nurse, $12.87; baccalaureate, $13.02; and graduate, $13.75. About half of the nursing staff were reported to be at the maximum hourly rate of pay. For the licensed practical nurse, starting hourly salaries were $7.75 on average and $9.07 maximum. The annual salary increase was on average 8.0% for 1988.

Benefit packages were provided by most hospices—26 of 29. The average value of the package for the registered nurse was 22% of salary; for the licensed practical nurse, 20%; and for the nursing assistant, 25%. About 40% (or 11) of the hospice employers did not provide retirement benefits for their employees. Most employers provided vacation, holiday, sick and personal leave, health and life insurance, and continuing education benefits.

For another indicator of the availability of nursing staff, hospice administrators were asked to comment on their ability to adhere to practice standards. Several reported they frequently or occasionally found that continuity of assignments, number of nursing hours for each patient, and patient satisfaction were affected unfavorably.

Some hospices reported they incurred overtime expense. Eleven agencies spent, on average, $6,654 for registered nurse overtime; five spent an average of $1,662 for licensed practical nurse overtime; and nine hospices spent an average of $600 for nursing assistant overtime. Not all hospices spent money for recruitment of nursing staff. Of the 29 hospices, however, 18 spent, on average, $5,041 for advertising; fewer indicated they incurred expenses for salaries and travel for recruitment. Of the 29, 18 hospices used temporary staff to supplement their permanent nursing personnel: 6 hospices indicated they obtained temporary personnel from an in-house staffing pool, and 13 hired temporary staff from freestanding staffing agencies. Three hospices reported their average annual expense for in-house pool nursing staff was $16,261 in 1988, while 13 hospices reported an annual average of $56,799 spent on temporary nursing staff from freestanding staffing agencies in 1988.

Thus our findings show relatively low vacancy and turnover rates for nursing staff in the hospice setting. While some expenses were incurred for overtime and temporary nursing personnel, it is not clear whether these strategies were used to accommodate fluctuations in caseloads. While salaries were relatively low, with little differential for advanced education, fringe benefits were competitive with other employment opportunities. It is well known that the hospice setting makes use of volunteer personnel. Our data do not capture this segment of the hospice staff and how the use of volunteers affects the employment and working conditions of the paid staff.

Discussion

The health services presented in this chapter—home health agencies, public health units, and hospices—are all community based and provide somewhat similar services. Here the similarities end.

Employees in the three agencies are a different mix of nursing personnel. Home health agencies rely on all three levels of nursing personnel: the registered nurse, licensed practical nurse, and the nursing assistant. In public health, more reliance on the registered nurse is seen in the ratios of nursing staff employed. The registered nurse is classified into clinic nurse, public health nurse, and nurse practitioner. This is the only setting dependent on the advanced practitioner category of nursing personnel. In the hospice setting, where many volunteers work, the registered nurse plays a key role.

Vacancy rates for the home health agency were by far the highest of the three community health service agencies studied. The high rates were apparent in all levels of nursing personnel. The hospice setting reported the lowest rates. In the home health setting, turnover rates were highest for the licensed practical nurse; in the hospice setting, turnover rates for nursing personnel were lowest for this category of staff. Turnover rates were not available for nurses in public health in 1988.

While salary information was not available for the nursing assistant, comparisons of RN and LPN salaries showed that the public health setting had the lowest rate of pay for both levels of staff. The home health agency setting reported the highest salary levels for both categories of nurses and thus may be a major competitor for nurses in the traditional public health setting. Salary increases were also highest for home health agency nurses and lowest for the public health nurse. Public health led both home health agencies and hospices in fringe benefit levels, however, although the home health agencies and hospices indicated the fringe benefits provided to the nursing assistant were higher than for other categories of nursing

TABLE 8.9 Comparison of Select Variables for Nursing Personnel in Home
Health Agencies, Public Health Units, and Hospices, 1988

Measure	Home Health Agency Average	Number	Public Health Unit Average	Number	Hospice Average	Number
FTE: nursing staff ratio						
RN	0.24	(196)	0.77	(67)	NA	
LPN	0.40	(141)	0.05	(67)	NA	
NA	0.37	(75)	0.17	(67)	NA	
FTE vacancy rate:						
RN	31.2	(80)	20.5	(67)	7.2	(29)
LPN	83.3	(110)	11.1	(67)	9.4	(11)
NA	44.5	(19)	11.9	(67)	9.3	(26)
FTE turnover:						
RN	51.9	(136)	NA		28.3	(23)
LPN	29.9	(64)	NA		54.6	(6)
NA	67.4	(33)	NA		33.8	(12)
Beginning hourly salary						
RN	$11.31	(155)	$8.32	(67)	$10.01	(25)
LPN	$9.18	(97)	$7.15	(67)	$7.75	(16)
NA	NA		NA		NA	
Annual increase salary:						
RN	9.0%	(121)	5.0%	(67)	9.4%	(26)
LPN	11.4%	(67)	5.6%	(67)	7.3%	(9)
NA	9.0%	(78)	4.3%	(67)	9.9%	(17)
Fringe benefit/salary:						
RN	20.6%	(131)	22.0%	(67)	22.0%	(29)
LPN	18.5%	(65)	22.0%	(67)	19.8%	(13)
NA	23.2%	(99)	20.0%	(67)	25.4%	(21)

personnel or than for nursing assistants in the public health setting.
Thus public health had better fringe benefit packages than the other
settings, but salaries were lower.

Community-based services are offered in the home and clinic settings. For home-based services provided by home health agencies,
hospices, and many health departments, a large proportion of the
clients are older persons. Much emphasis has been placed on providing home-based care for older persons in lieu of more restrictive
institutional care. Because of the growing proportion of older persons, particularly functionally impaired over-85-year-olds, expansion of community and home-based services will occur in the future
(Kane & Kane, 1987; Serow, Cowart, & Chen, 1990).

Finally, examination of nursing personnel in community-based services demonstrates working conditions for nurses in profit and not-for-profit health care industries. For the most part, home health agencies are owned by proprietary firms (63%), while 33% are under not-for-profit ownership and 4% are publicly owned. On the other hand, all hospices were nonprofit, and public health agencies were owned by the county, with supplemental state funding. Further underscoring the proprietary nature of the home health agency industry, 18.5% of the agencies studied were part of national chains, while none of the hospices had such an affiliation. In a sense, public health agencies could be considered part of a state-wide firm with a strong county government influence.

In terms of for-profit firms, nurses fared better in the home health industry in terms of salaries, although the fringe benefit package did not have as much value as those benefits in public health. As public agencies, public health units reported lower turnover despite lower salaries. Such stability may have been due to the state personnel system and more valuable benefits program, including a generous retirement plan. Public health personnel were also unionized, something that had not occurred among the privately owned home health and hospice industries. The hospices representing the not-for-profit sector had lower salaries and benefits programs than the profit-dominated home health agency industry. Thus nurses electing to work in the public health units earned lower salaries but had more job security and retirement benefits. Nurses in the corporate home health agencies had higher salaries but greater potential for turnover. In the hospice setting, nurses earned salaries that were below those in home health agencies but were greater than those in public health. Benefits were comparable with other privately owned health services, but not as great as in the public sector.

NINE

Supplemental Nursing Staff

MARIE E. COWART

DIANNE L. SPEAKE

As nursing personnel became scarce during 1986 and 1987, the hospital and nursing home industries in Florida publicly expressed concern about the amount of funds spent on supplemental nursing staff. Anecdotal reports from health care facilities indicated that the provision of supplemental staffing services had expanded in an effort to meet the increased demand for nursing personnel in a time of nursing shortage. As a result of the concerns of the hospital and nursing home industry, Florida Statute Chapter 88-394 was passed by the legislature and included a section authorizing the study of

> the impact of the labor shortage on the increased use of temporary nursing pool agencies by institutional providers; the influence of this trend on the availability, quality and costs of services provided; and the costs and benefits of potential regulation of such nursing pool agencies in light of the shortage.

This chapter will examine the findings from the study on employment and use of nursing personnel in staffing agencies in Florida. For the purpose of the study, a *supplemental staffing agency* (SSA) is defined as "an agency or organization that supplies licensed and nonlicensed nursing staff and contracts with clients such as hospitals, nursing homes and other health facilities to provide nursing staff for temporary or supplemental assignments." The chapter is organized into four sections: overview of the issues, methodology, findings, and conclusions.

Overview of the Issues

Supplemental staffing agencies have come into the limelight recently. They are a new version of an old form of service: nurse registries. In the past, nurse registries served as a clearinghouse, putting nurse and patient together to contract for services with monies for services exchanged directly between the patient and the nurse. In return, the nurse paid a fee to the agency for placement. In contrast, the freestanding proprietary SSAs of today still place private duty nurses, but the agency bills the patient. In addition, SSAs, most of which began in the 1970s, provide nurses for hospitals and nursing homes and also contract with state agencies to provide services for group homes for the developmentally disabled, prison health services, or children's medical service clinics.

Kehrer and Szapiro's (1984) national study of randomly selected temporary staffing services estimated that some 1,300 to 1,600 were active in 1981, with the majority (97.9%) indicating that they were for-profit entities providing RN, LPN, CNA, and orderly staff. Three quarters were located in just 15 states; 3 states—California, Florida, and New York—had more than 100 offices. Agencies had, on average, eight institutional clients—five hospitals and three nursing homes—and an average of 61 RNs on contract. During this same year, the National Commission on Nursing (1981) identified supplementary staffing as a nursing practice option.

For nurses, the SSA provides opportunities for flexibility in work schedule and choice of assignment, although full-time employment is not guaranteed because demands for staffing nurses vary. Inherent in SSA employment is the absence of structure and affiliation with an organization that has a specific goal in the patient care provided. For nurses wanting to supplement their salary and work independently, SSA employment provides a higher hourly rate of pay, but without benefits.

Kehrer, Deiman, and Szapiro's (1984) survey of SSA registered nurse employees and institutional clients revealed that the most attractive aspects of SSA employment for RNs were the flexible days and hours of work. Other reasons given as important were higher hourly wages, extra income, preference not to have a full-time job, and the desire to avoid "hospital politics." Lesser reasons included accommodating family responsibilities and attending school. Of the RN respondents, 40% had worked for more than one agency during the previous 12 months even though they worked only part-time. Respondents reported being assigned as a staff or charge nurse in hospitals, assigned as treatment/medication or charge nurse in nursing homes, assigned to settings where they had previous assignments, and working weekends, evening, and night shifts. Most reported they did not have a long-term commitment to SSA work, with more nurses moving to permanent employment than to part-time work with an SSA agency.

As early as 1977, Jett cited the use of supplemental nursing personnel as a hospital cost control measure (1977). Coss (1989) later posited that SSAs exist because the market demanded them to create competition. This was accomplished when the agency allowed the hospital to maintain a minimal nursing staff suited to the average daily patient census. When increased census required increased nursing staff, supplemental personnel were obtained from the local staffing agency. Thus hospitals minimized the number of underused staff on the payroll during periods of low census, resulting in variable nurse labor costs rather than a fixed expense item. Coss also proposed that agency staffing provides a "market answer" to the intrinsic sluggishness of nursing wages due to the monopsonistic character of the hospital industry, which is the major employer of nurses.

For nursing homes, another situation occurred regarding the use of supplemental staffing largely because of the traditionally more stable year-round patient census and the fixed level of Medicaid reimbursement. Nursing homes with a stable census used supplemental staffing to fill vacant positions due to shortage of personnel and temporary vacancies due to absences of regular staff. Both of these causes lend themselves to corrections in personnel policies by the nursing home. In recent years, however, Florida nursing home patient censuses fluctuated similarly to those of Florida hospitals (Florida Health Care Cost Containment Board, 1989a). Nursing homes that experienced cyclical variations in patient census also experienced efficiencies in labor costs for nurses by using supplemental nursing staff.

Florida's procompetitive regulatory environment, coupled with the implementation of the federal prospective payment system, helped to provide incentives for the expansion of supplemental nursing staffing services in Florida during 1985-1988. The McKnight Task Force on Competition and Consumer Choices in Health Care, established in 1983, emphasized the need to provide incentives for competition in the health care marketplace in Florida. The Task

Force—comprising 21 representatives of the hospital, insurance, and business industries as well as public policymakers, physicians, public health administrators, and advocates of the elderly and medically indigent—opposed adoption of a rate-setting approach to health cost containment. Instead, the Task Force recommended that specific price competition and market forces be encouraged in Florida. The current state of Florida's health care marketplace is largely a result of this philosophical approach to health policy.

The Florida Health Care Association and Florida Association of Homes for the Aged (1987) responded to the increased growth in supplemental nursing personnel by surveying the 450 nursing homes in Florida during 1987. The 261 respondents reported they spent $3.7 million for temporary agency/nurse pool personnel during the July 1 through September 30 quarter. Hourly rates for agency nursing personnel were approximately double the salaries paid to permanent employees. Evening and night shifts were reported to be the most affected.

In the following year, the Florida Hospital Association (1989) surveyed 68 of the member acute care hospitals regarding the use of SSAs: 72% of responding hospitals indicated they used SSAs at a rate of 246.6 hours per week, or 6.2 FTEs. Critical care and medical-surgical nursing units were the most frequently cited areas where staffing nurses were assigned. The RN and LPN categories of personnel were most frequently used.

The Florida Health Care Cost Containment Board (Serow, Cowart, & Chen, 1990) survey of hospitals, nursing homes, and home health agencies reported that, in 1988, Florida hospitals spent an average of $570,000 for SSA staff while nursing homes averaged $91,400. In addition, 80% of hospitals, 67% of nursing homes, and 28% of home health agencies in the HCCCB study sample reported they used temporary staff from either outside SSAs or internal in-house staffing pools.

The literature documents a number of issues and concerns about use of SSAs (Eggland, 1989; Long, 1984; Regan, 1981, 1982; Sheridan, Bronstein, & Walker, 1982). These issues range from concerns about the nursing practices of temporary staff to liability for staff injuries. Nursing practice issues included inexperience, medication errors, and lack of continuity. Personnel and agency issues included lateness or cancellations, prescreening of agency applicants, little orientation, evaluation of temporary nurses, checking licensure status, on-the-job injury of agency nurse, and mobility of unacceptable nurses from one agency to another.

More recent literature seems to demonstrate that many of these concerns have been addressed by both the industry and the hospital association (Korman, 1988; Sharp, 1989). For example, the 1980 Joint Commission on the Accreditation of Healthcare Organizations (JCAHO) standards required hospitals using SSAs to develop contracts that clearly outline agency and hospital responsibilities, agreed-on rates, and orientation and evaluation procedures (Long, 1984; Robertson, 1987; Sheridan et al., 1982). More important, the standards opened communication between institution and agency.

Among hospitals, a private sector approach is evolving as hospitals in Florida and other states are creating preferred provider arrangements with select SSAs ("Hospital-Agency Pacts," 1989). Contracts, which may last only six months, are between one or more hospitals and one or more agencies to establish prices and exclusivity in doing business. A federal judge in Florida, however, has responded in a suit brought by other staffing agencies that such contracts violate antitrust laws because more than 35% of the market will be controlled ("ANA Fights Cap," 1989; "Hospitals Try New Tactic," 1989).

Both industry and professional news media have found supplemental staffing to be a viable topic. The higher costs of agency nurses has led the nursing home industry in Massachusetts and eight other states to seek legislation to cap rates and set standards for agency use ("Hospitals Try New Tactic," 1989; "Massachusetts Moves to Limit," 1989). Under leadership of the American Health Care Association, an organization representing for-profit nursing homes, legislation aimed at reducing Medicaid expenditures by setting maximum rates charged for agency nurses was introduced in several states. The nursing home industry contends that the agency nurse costs are double the starting salaries paid by the homes, while agencies say nurses are paid 65 cents on the billing dollar with the rest covering expenses such as taxes, insurance, and overhead. Profit is reported to be 4%-5%.

Massachusetts was the first state to pass rate-setting legislation. In most states, with the exception of Massachusetts and Tennessee, hospital groups have not entered the debate, and state nurse associations have opposed such legislation. A new enterprise, independent referral entities, which places nurses as independent contractors, is in turn being opposed by the now traditional SSAs. Since November 1988, Massachusetts agencies have had their rates limited, although nurse salaries are not restricted. Under agency pay, nurses make about 35% more than institutional staff nurses, but, because they are not paid benefits, adjustments for about 20% to 30% of wages must be made to account for fringe benefits ("Nursing Home Industry," 1988).

In Florida, a bill was passed providing for the regulation of nursing pools by the Department of Business Regulation (DBR), which include any person, firm, corporation, partnership, or association engaged for hire in the business of providing temporary employment in health care facilities for medical personnel including, without limitation, nurses, nursing assistants, nurse aides, and orderlies. The statute, however, excludes nursing registries, independent nurse contractors, and agencies licensed as home health agencies under Florida Statutes Chapter 400. The effect of this law has been minimal, with only 58 agencies registered with the DBR in 1989.

Methodology

The purpose of the study was to answer major questions asked in the legislative mandate for the study. Questionnaires were developed in fall 1989 with the assistance of the Nursing Shortage Study Technical Advisory Panel and were approved by the Florida Health Care Cost Containment Board. They included items on the following subjects areas:

- organization and structure of the supplemental staffing agency
- kinds of clients served by the supplemental staffing agency
- characteristics of contracts between clients and agencies
- number of and charges for services offered by agencies
- categories of personnel hired by agencies and their number, preparation, wages, and benefits
- policies for orientation, supervision, and evaluation as well as handling substance abusers
- pre- and postagency employment trends
- use of travel/contract staff
- other agency expense items

Lists of SSAs in Florida were developed by obtaining names and addresses from known staffing agencies from the Florida Health Care Cost Containment Board, the Bureau of Business Regulation, and the telephone books of the 15 largest cities in the state. The 744 questionnaires were sent by certified mail to staffing agencies in December 1989. Board staff conducted a preliminary review of returned questionnaires and obtained additional responses by telephone inquiries of study participants.

Analysis of the data was complicated by several factors. First, agencies provided a wide variety and mix of services. Second, SSAs used many configurations for maintaining business records (e.g., types of services, numbers of clients, and numbers of staff). Third, some reports were submitted for multiple office sites. The use of a follow-up telephone interview clarified responses and corrected many of these problems. When reports were identified for multiple offices, these cases were dropped from the analysis. Other known inconsistencies will be identified with the reporting of the findings.

Findings

This section reports the responses to the questionnaires by participating agencies. Findings are organized into a description of the sample, the clients of temporary staffing agencies, the services offered, the employees of agencies, revenues and expenses of agencies, and, finally, a description of several miscellaneous topics related to temporary staffing agencies.

SAMPLE

The total number of SSAs surveyed was 744. Of the questionnaires sent to them, 97 were returned undelivered by the post office; 128 were not returned; and 269 respondents indicated they did not provide nursing personnel to health care facilities at the time of the survey. A total of 197 SSAs and 7 agencies that placed contract/travel nurses constituted the sample. The findings of this chapter will be limited to the 197 responding SSAs.

Of the 197 respondents, 4 had been established prior to 1965, although none had provided supplemental nursing staffing services at that time. The majority (95%) of agencies were established after 1970,

TABLE 9.1 Select Characteristics of Sample of Florida Supplemental
Staffing Agencies by Year, 1989

Year	Year Established		Year Began Temporary Staffing Services	
	Number	*Percentage*	*Number*	*Percentage*
Before 1965	4	2.0	0	0.0
1965-1969	6	3.0	2	1.0
1970-1974	33	16.8	30	15.2
1975-1979	27	13.7	28	14.2
1980-1984	29	14.7	30	15.2
1985-1989	92	46.7	102	51.8
Missing data	6	3.1	5	2.6
Total	197	100.0	197	100.0

with almost half beginning business between 1985 and 1989 (Table 9.1).
Approximately half (49.2%) of the SSAs were classified as independent
corporations; the remainder indicated they were owned by another corporate entity. The most common structural arrangement was ownership in a multiagency system not affiliated with a hospital (37%). Other
arrangements included single-entity for-profit agency (8.0%), for-profit
subsidiary of a not-for-profit hospital (6.0%), ownership by a general
personnel agency (5.0%), and ownership by a not-for-profit multihospi-
tal system (3.0%). No agencies indicated they were wholly voluntary or
publicly owned; one was nonprofit. Respondents represented all geographic areas of the state with greatest concentrations of SSAs in the
Tampa-St. Petersburg (25%), Miami-Fort Lauderdale (23%), Orlando
(10%), Palm Beach (9%), Fort Myers (9%) areas, with fewer respondents
in the large northern Panhandle region (13%).

AGENCY CLIENTS

Agencies were asked to report the number of health facility clients
with whom they did business in 1988 and 1989. Hospitals received
services from the largest number of agencies. When comparing 1988
with 1989, agencies also showed the greatest increase in hospital
clients over other kinds of health care clients. Just under half of the
SSAs provided staff for hospitals in 1988, increasing to nearly 60%
of agencies in 1989. Other clients that frequently received staffing

TABLE 9.2 Select Characteristics of Sample of Florida Supplemental Staffing Agencies by District, 1989

DHRS District	Number	Percentage
District 1—Pensacola	1	0.5
District 2—Tallahassee	3	1.5
District 3—Gainesville	8	4.1
District 4—Jacksonville	14	7.1
District 5—St. Petersburg	32	16.3
District 6—Tampa	17	8.6
District 7—Orlando	20	10.1
District 8—Fort Myers	18	9.1
District 9—West Palm Beach	18	9.1
District 10—Fort Lauderdale	22	11.2
District 11—Miami	23	11.7
Missing data (out of state)	21	10.7
Total	197	100.0

services from agencies were nursing homes (increasing from 49% to 54% of agencies), home-based private duty (increasing from 40% to 48% of agencies), intermittent home health agency visits (increasing from 26% to 32% of agencies), and adult congregate living facilities (increasing from 29% to 35% of agencies; see Tables 9.2 and 9.3).

In 1989, staffing agencies had an average of 7.4 hospital clients, 8.6 nursing home clients, 3.7 adult congregate living facility clients, 5.8 physician office clients, 4.4 psychiatric inpatient unit clients (non-hospital based), 3.1 psychiatric outpatient facility clients, 1.9 health maintenance organization clients, 3.4 ambulatory surgical center clients, 1.8 hospice clients, 18.1 county health unit clients, and 2.3 ICFMR clients. On average, agencies provided services to 126.5 private individuals in their homes in 1989. They also conducted an average of 78.5 intermittent home visits through licensed home health agencies (Table 9.3).

Discussions with agency staff during telephone interviews revealed that many of the services to psychiatric inpatient units, county health units, hospices, and other settings consisted of home visit services. This may have accounted for the large response for county health unit clients, which likely represented patients rather than county health units. Other settings where nursing staff were

TABLE 9.3 Types and Numbers of Clients Provided Services by Sample Florida Temporary Staffing Agencies, 1988 and 1989 ($n = 197$)

Category of Services	1988			1989		
	Do Not Provide	Do Provide	Average Number Clients	Do Not Provide	Do Provide	Average Number Clients
Acute care hospital	103	94	6.8	84	113	7.4
Nursing home	101	88*	7.3	91	106	8.6
Private duty home visits**	115	79	103.5	102	95	126.5
Intermittent home visits for home health agency**	145	52	86.0	133	64	78.5
Adult congregate living facility (ACLF)	139	58	3.7	129	68	2.5
Physician's office	159	38	8.6	150	47	5.8
Psychiatric inpatient, non-hospital based**	166	31	2.4	158	39	4.4
Psychiatric outpatient facility**	189	7	1.7	187	10	3.1
Health maintenance organization	183	14	2.5	175	22	1.9
Ambulatory surgical center	184	13	3.2	181	16	3.4
Hospice**	162	35	1.5	164	33	1.8
County health unit**	190	7	1.4	182	15	1.8
ICFMR***	189	8	2.5	188	9	2.3

*Eight nursing homes reporting state or national data were omitted.
**Most services were likely to be home visits.
***ICFMR is intermediate care for the mentally retarded.

assigned included group homes, correctional facilities, and day-care centers.

Information about the volume of services was obtained by determining the average number of hours of services provided during the week of December 4-10, 1989: 77 agencies provided an average of 500 hours of registered nurse services to hospitals, with critical care units receiving the largest amount of services. Only seven agencies provided pediatric services, and ten placed registered nurses in operating rooms of hospitals. Hours of nursing assistant services were one third those of registered nurses for hospitals. In contrast, agencies provided five times as many nursing assistant as registered nurse hours to nursing homes during the reporting week, although only 50 agencies provided these services. Placement of

TABLE 9.4 Average Number of Hours of Nursing Services to Hospitals, Nursing Homes, and In-Home Care, per Reporting Temporary Staffing Agency in Florida, December 4–10, 1989

Range and Number of Services	Do Not Provide	Do Provide	Hours of Service Average	SD
Hospital:				
Total registered nurse services	117	77	500.0	1221.5
medical-surgical	138	56	141.8	305.2
critical care	146	48	226.1	277.9
operating room	184	10	103.9	156.2
emergency room	175	19	121.2	168.6
obstetrics/newborn	179	15	84.1	122.9
pediatrics	187	7	136.4	186.4
psychiatry	176	18	80.0	98.2
Total LPN services	136	58	192.3	214.9
medical-surgical	146	48	166.4	187.5
critical care	177	17	119.9	169.9
Total nursing assistant services	157	37	145.8	206.5
Other	172	22	165.0	240.7
Nursing home:				
Total registered nurse services	172	22	64.4	95.8
Total LPN services	154	40	219.8	428.4
Total nursing assistant services	144	50	302.6	882.2
Home health:				
Total registered nurse services	145	49	93.6	136.1
Total LPN services	144	50	134.0	129.6
Total home aide services	123	71	535.7	527.9
Total sitter services	180	14	91.6	170.1
Total companion services	169	25	182.5	249.6

home health aides through home health agencies was the largest category of service, with 536 average hours provided by the 71 agencies that reported this service (Table 9.4).

Only 10% of agencies reported an absence of contracts with clients. Liability insurance requirements were included in 81% of agency contracts. Other content commonly included in written contracts between agencies and their clients concerned qualifications of personnel, 79%; orientation process, 79%; verification of license, 77%; scheduling policies, 74%; cancellation terms, 74%; and supervision and evaluation process, 72% (Table 9.5). The contents of these agency contracts often varied according to the preferences of clients.

TABLE 9.5 Frequency of Items Included in Contracts Between Sample Florida Temporary Staffing Agencies and Their Clients, 1989 (*n* = 197)

Item	Frequency Number	Percentage
Liability insurance requirements	157	80.9
Qualifications of personnel	153	78.9
Orientation process	155	78.7
Verification of license	150	77.3
Scheduling policies and practices	146	74.1
Terms for cancellation	143	73.7
Supervision process	141	72.7
Evaluation process	139	71.6
Screening tests for personnel	132	68.0
Wage charge	134	68.0
Skills checklist	130	67.0
CPR certification requirements	133	67.5
Policies on disciplinary procedures	123	63.4
Noncompetition clause for recruitment of personnel	123	63.4
Infection control policies	122	62.9
Medication procedures	119	61.3
Cancellation penalties	119	61.3
Discounts for volume	102	52.6
Discounts for early payment	85	43.8
Discounts for early scheduling	78	40.2
Other	22	11.3

AGENCY PERSONNEL

Well over half of the agencies in the sample employed registered nurses (68%), licensed practical nurses (65%), and nursing assistants (59%) for placement in their clients' settings. Companions (31%), homemakers (26%), physical therapists/technicians (29%), occupational therapists (24%), and social workers (22%) were other common categories of employees hired for placement with clients (Table 9.6). One agency specialized in placing allied health personnel such as respiratory therapists and radiology technicians and did not place nursing staff. A large proportion of agency services in this study were directed at placing personnel in patients' homes.

Some information about the characteristics of registered nurses hired by temporary staffing agencies was obtained, although less than

TABLE 9.6 Categories of Personnel Hired by Sample Florida
Temporary Staffing Agencies, 1989 (n = 197)

Categories of Personnel	Do Not Employ	Do Employ	Number of Employees Average	SD
Registered nurse	63	134	61.4	85.7
Graduate nurse (GN)	193	4	5.3	3.3
Licensed practical nurse	68	129	48.6	65.8
Graduate practical nurse	192	5	58.0	86.7
Nursing assistant	81	116	79.0	82.3
Orderly	176	21	30.0	93.4
Homemaker	146	51	16.5	30.2
Companion	135	62	13.3	29.1
Sitter	158	39	12.4	16.7
Physical therapist/tech	141	56	4.3	4.4
Occupational therapist	151	47	1.8	1.2
Social worker	154	43	1.9	1.3
Respiratory therapist/tech	168	29	9.5	25.9
Mental health technician	183	14	10.0	12.5
Registered dietitian	183	14	1.1	0.3
Unit secretary/clerk	189	8	8.8	16.8
Advanced registered nurse practitioner	191	6	3.0	3.5
Radiology technician	193	4	11.5	12.0
Medical doctor	194	3	1.7	1.2
Pharmacist	195	2	1.5	0.7
Psychologist	196	1	1.0	0.0
Certified nurse midwife	196	1	2.0	0.0
Nurse anesthetist	196	1	1.0	0.0
Physician's assistant	196	1	2.0	0.0

half of the responding agencies provided this information. From those that did respond: 41% of registered nurses were prepared in associate degree nursing programs, 28% in diploma programs, 25% in baccalaureate programs, and 6% had graduate degrees (Table 9.7). Comparison of educational preparation of nurses in hospitals, nursing homes, and home health agencies showed that agency nurses had more educational preparation than nurses employed in other settings.

Data on the age of the registered nurse indicated that agencies employed relatively large numbers of nurses who were under the

TABLE 9.7 Select Characteristics of Registered Nurses in Sample of Florida Temporary Staffing Agencies, 1989

Characteristic	Percentage	Responses
Educational preparation:		
associate degree	41.1	(100)
diploma	28.3	(97)
baccalaureate	24.5	(96)
master's degree	4.4	(43)
doctorate	1.7	(6)
Total	100.0	
Age of RN employed, 1989:		
less than 25 years	12.0	(46)
25-34 Years	31.3	(93)
35-44 years	26.1	(94)
45-54 years	12.4	(80)
55-64 years	7.0	(57)
65 and over	11.2	(26)
Total	100.0	
Length of employment:		
less than 1 year	28.5	(99)
2 to 5 years	35.3	(103)
6 to 10 years	15.7	(42)
11 to 20 years	9.1	(17)
more than 20 years	11.4	(4)
Total	100.0	

NOTE: These are weighted percentages based on the number of responses in each cell.

age of 25 years or over the age of 55 compared with other health care employers. Agency nurses were employed varying lengths of time: 28% for less than one year, 35% for one to five years, 16% for six to ten years, and 21% for more than ten years (Table 9.7).

Recruitment and retention methods used by agencies included media advertising (80%), incentives to current staff to recruit (69%), bonus after minimum number of shifts worked (54%), and sign-on bonus (50%). Three quarters of the reporting agencies required the personnel they hired to have previous recent (within three years) hospital experience prior to placement in hospitals.

SSAs estimated that the majority of employees were recruited from within the same county (67%) and had been previously employed by either a local hospital (52%) or another staffing agency (50%). Other previous employers included a local home health agency (36%), local nursing home (21%), or local physician's office (8%). One third of agency employees were reported to be recruited from out of county and 23% from out of state. Agencies estimated that 56% of registered nurses and licensed practical nurses held jobs in another staffing agency, about one third in a local hospital, and one fifth in a local nursing home.

The majority of agencies reported that nurses preferred to work for agencies because of flexible work scheduling (81%) and higher pay per hour (60%). Some indicated that nurses liked the choice of assignment, experience gained by working in a variety of settings, and right to refuse an assignment. Independence and autonomy in the work was mentioned, particularly in relation to making home visits or providing private duty services and giving direct patient care. Others indicated that nurses joined agency staff to get away from institutional politics and because they felt overworked and "burned out" from staff shortages and too much overtime. Others worked on agency staffs because they preferred part-time work with no weekends, allowing more time with family or completion of education. Some used the agency for employment when new to an area until they found a full-time position or as a second job to supplement income. Other liked being paid daily or weekly and, for some, agency work provided satisfaction and fit their life-style at the time (Table 9.8).

Not enough work to guarantee 40 hours employment weekly was the major reason employers gave for nurses leaving agency work (62%). Needing fringe benefits, particularly health insurance, was the reason mentioned second most frequently (40%). Many agencies reported that nurses left agency work to work full-time in hospitals or other health care settings offering better salaries and job security. Some nurses wanted the support system provided by working with others in a structured setting, more continuity, or a management position. Others left employment with the agency because of moving away from the area, wanting to retire or to leave nursing, or for other personal reasons. Some left to work with another agency that offered a higher salary or because they learned that the current agency was losing a contract with a facility where they were usually assigned. Some tired of home visits, disliked the paperwork associated with home health

TABLE 9.8 Agency Opinions Regarding Reasons Registered Nurses
Preferred Agency Employment in Florida, 1989 (*n* = 197)

Reason for Agency Employment	Number	Percentage
Flexible work schedule	158	81.4
Higher pay per hour	116	59.8
Choice of assignment		
and variety of settings	75	38.7
Independence/autonomy	19	9.8
Like private duty, direct patient care	17	8.8
No institutional politics	15	7.7
New to area, use agency		
to locate full-time job	12	6.2
Income supplement to primary job	11	5.7
Felt overworked due to		
short staff, burnout	10	5.2
Like respect shown by agency staff	10	5.2
Want part-time, no weekends	9	4.7
Like daily or weekly paycheck	9	4.7
Like shift differential and bonus	5	2.6
Work in agency while between jobs	3	1.5
Satisfaction with agency work	3	1.5
Fits life-style	2	1.0
Allows more time with family	1	0.5

NOTE: Percentages do not add to 100 because of multiple responses.

agency home visits, feared going into dangerous areas, or had difficulty with transportation for home visiting (Table 9.9).

EMPLOYMENT POLICIES

Agencies reported on preemployment screening factors and on procedures for orientation, supervision, and evaluation of their employees. There were nearly universal prescreening procedures by agencies for references, license, and skills as well as health screening. Other frequently included items in the preemployment screening process were health history, cardiopulmonary resuscitation certification, medication proficiency testing, and verification of specialty certification (Table 9.10).

Agencies were asked to provide information about orientation, supervision, and evaluation of staffing employees. Only 11% provided more than eight hours of orientation, while 6% provided no orientation

NURSES IN THE WORKPLACE

TABLE 9.9 Agency Opinions Regarding Reasons Registered Nurses Leave Agency Employment in Florida, 1989 (n = 197)

Reason for Leaving Agency Employment	Number	Percentage
Not enough work to guarantee 40 hours weekly	120	61.9
Need fringe benefits	78	40.2
Move away from the area	40	20.6
To go full-time with hospital or other setting with better salary and job security	29	14.9
Higher salary	18	9.3
Personal reasons	10	5.2
Want continuity, tired of variety of assignments	8	4.1
Go to work for another agency	8	4.1
Want to leave nursing	6	3.1
Burnout as an agency nurse	5	2.6
Too much paperwork associated with home care	5	2.6
Inadequate pay	4	2.1
Lack of support system, too independent	4	2.1
Difficulties with transportation	4	2.1
Do not like agency policies, poor organization	3	1.5
Retirement	2	1.0
Tired of going into dangerous areas for home care	2	1.0
Terminated by agency	1	0.5
Assignments were canceled	1	0.5
Do not like working in ICFMR	1	0.5
Want to return to management position	1	0.5

NOTE: Percentages do not add to 100 because of multiple responses.

at all. Four agencies reported that they placed nurses in hospitals without some form of orientation, but none reported an absence of orientation prior to nursing home placement. Most agencies provided facility-specific orientation or negotiated with the facility for joint orientation. Similarly, more than half of the agencies provided on-site supervision of agency staff on request of the facility where agency employees were placed. Three fourths of agencies solicited facility evaluation of agency nurses with agency follow-up and licensure and specialty credential

TABLE 9.10 Preemployment Screening Factors for Sample of Florida Supplemental Staffing Agencies, 1989 (*n* = 197)

Item	Yes Number	%	No Number	%	Plan To Number	%
Reference check	193	98	4	2	0	0
Licensure check	192	97	5	3	0	0
Skills checklist	189	96	5	3	3	1
Health screening tests	189	96	5	3	3	1
Health history	184	93	13	7	0	0
Current CPR certification	175	90	18	8	4	2
Medication proficiency test	171	87	23	12	2	1
Documentation of handicaps	157	20	35	18	3	2
Verify specialty certification	170	87	20	10	5	3
Specialty testing for specialty assignment	145	76	43	22	3	2
Continuing education records	142	73	42	22	10	5
Police record check	139	72	50	24	7	4

verification. Agencies reported that three fourths of hospitals and nursing homes allowed on-site evaluation visits by agency office staff and that less than three fourths of these facilities returned written evaluations of agency nurses (Tables 9.11 and 9.12).

To detect potential substance abusers, 87.6% of agencies verified previous employment and licensure history of applicants, and more than 90% reported evidence of substance abuse to the Board of Nursing. One third of agencies referred nurses with substance abuse problems to employee assistance programs (Tables 9.11 and 9.12).

AGENCY REVENUES AND EXPENSES

Table 9.13 summarizes the average hourly pay for categories of nursing personnel in hospital, nursing home, and home care by regular daytime, shift, weekend, holidays, and specialty assignments. Holiday pay was reported by a number of agencies to be at the rate of time and a half of daytime pay levels, although this does not appear to be the case for all agencies because the average for all reporting agencies is one-and-one-third average daytime salary.

TABLE 9.11 Characteristics of Orientation, Supervision, and Evaluation of Employees in Sample of Florida Temporary Staffing Agencies, 1989 (*n* = 197)

Characteristic	Number	Percentage
Orientation of new staff:		
8 hours or less including preemployment testing	90	45.7
8 hours or less excluding preemployment testing	65	33.0
More than 8 hours of orientation including preemployment testing	14	7.1
More than 8 hours of orientation excluding preemployment testing	8	4.1
Other	9	4.6
None	11	5.6
Work setting orientation for new staff (more than one choice):		
Agency provides general information, facility provides specific	122	61.9
Negotiate orientation by facility and agency jointly	102	51.7
Negotiate orientation by facility on individual basis	96	48.7
1-2 shifts in assigned work setting with on-site agency instructor	19	9.6
More than 2 shifts in assigned work settings with on-site agency instructor	5	2.5
None, orientation is facility responsibility	6	3.0
Agency supervisory responsibilities for employee performance in facility:		
Agency provides supervisory support on request of facility	117	59.4
Contracting facility assumes all responsibility for supervision	73	37.1
Agency provides on-site supervision of agency nurses at all times	25	12.7
Agency provides direct supervision during orientation only	8	4.1
Agency methods for monitoring quality of care by agency employees:		
Agency nurse evaluations completed by client with agency follow-up	154	78.2
Agency nurse evaluations completed by client with no agency follow-up	10	5.1
On-site quality audits conducted by agency with agency follow-up	110	55.8

TABLE 9.11 Continued

Characteristic	Number	Percentage
Specialty credentialing/experience		
requirements prior to assignments	141	71.6
Licensure monitoring	147	74.6
None	2	1.0
Other	35	17.8
Methods used to detect or track substance abuse among agency nurse staff:		
Preemployment drug screening only	3	1.5
Preemployment and periodic		
drug screening with follow-up		
of positive tests	3	1.5
Review employment/licensure		
history as part of preemployment		
reference checks	173	87.8
Employee assistance programs		
for abusers	64	32.5
None	13	6.6
Other	13	6.6

Development of estimates to compare hospital, nursing home, and agency pay levels for nursing staff was complicated by the fact that the most recent available hospital and nursing home salary data were for 1988 while agency data were for 12 months later in 1989. The average beginning hourly salary for the hospital employed registered nurse (RN) was $10.31 in 1988. Adding 25.2% for fringe benefits and 8.5% average annual salary increase, the hospital nurse average beginning hourly salary in 1989 was estimated to be $13.99 per hour in 1989. Maximum hourly salary range for the registered nurse in the hospital for daytime hours was $12.11 in 1988, or $16.45 per hour including fringe benefits worth 25.2% of salary and 8.5% annual salary increase. This compares with an average $18.21 hourly wage earned by the agency RN assigned to the hospital in the same year (Serow & Cowart, 1990). For RNs employed in nursing homes, comparable figures are $12.13 (average beginning hourly salary), $13.27 (maximum), and $16.04 (agency).

Similarly, the licensed practical nurse (LPN) in Florida hospitals had an average beginning hourly salary of $7.20 in 1988, fringe benefits of 25.8%, and an average annual raise of 9%. Hospital hourly

TABLE 9.12 Select Agency Nurse Evaluation Practices by Florida Agencies and Their Clients, 1988

Practice	Number	Percentage
Agency notifies clients of nurses history of substance abuse (*n* = 192)	65	33.9
Agency reports evidence of substance abuse to Board of Nursing (*n* = 195)	176	90.3
Written periodic evaluations of agency staff completed by agency (*n* = 196)	176	89.8
Proportion of nursing home agency clients returning agency nurse evaluations (*n* = 99)	69	69.5
Proportion of hospital clients returning agency nurse evaluations (*n* = 118)	88	74.6
Percentage of nursing home clients allowing on-site quality audit by agency (*n* = 99)	74	74.4
Percentage of hospital clients allowing on-site quality audit by agency (*n* = 103)	73	70.7

salary and benefits for 1989 were estimated to be $11.65 for the licensed practical nurse compared with an average $15.19 hourly wage earned by the agency LPN assigned to the hospital in the same year (Serow & Cowart, 1990). For LPNs in nursing homes, average salaries were $10.51 for those employed directly versus $13.67 for agency employees.

The nursing assistant in Florida hospitals had an average beginning hourly salary of $4.64 in 1988, fringe benefits of 26.1%, and an average annual raise of 7.4%. Hospital hourly salary and benefits for 1989 were estimated to be $6.28 for the nursing assistant compared with an average hourly wage of $7.31 earned by the agency nursing assistant assigned to the hospital in the same year (Serow & Cowart, 1990). In nursing homes, those rates were $6.08 and $7.21, respectively.

Benefits were not provided to the employees of temporary staffing agencies by 75% of agencies in the sample. Although 108 agencies (56%) reported they provided more than the mandatory benefits (e.g., workman's compensation) to agency employees, only 44 agencies reported benefits in the amount of 20.96% of salary to registered nurses, 39 reported providing 22.95% to licensed practical nurses, and

TABLE 9.13 Average Charges and Expenses for Services by Sample Florida Temporary Staffing Agencies, December 4-10, 1989

Category Personnel	Average Hourly Charge for Service Dollar Amount	N	Average Hourly Pay to Employees Dollar Amount	N	Estimated Difference Dollar Amount	%
Hospital RN service:						
Medical-surgical—						
day	27.17	(114)	18.20	(98)	8.97	33.0
evening	27.97	(113)	18.88	(97)	9.09	32.5
night	28.57	(114)	19.33	(96)	9.24	32.3
weekend, day	29.23	(114)	19.54	(96)	9.69	33.2
holiday, day	36.25	(92)	24.84	(82)	11.41	31.5
Critical care—						
day	32.36	(113)	21.67	(91)	10.69	33.0
evening	33.26	(112)	22.62	(95)	10.64	32.0
night	33.80	(112)	22.26	(95)	11.54	34.1
weekend, day	34.71	(111)	23.37	(94)	11.34	32.7
holiday, day	43.31	(92)	28.83	(85)	14.48	33.4
OR, day	32.43	(61)	21.68	(53)	10.75	33.1
ER, day	32.77	(76)	22.52	(64)	10.25	31.3
Hospital LPN services:						
Medical-surgical—						
day	21.36	(108)	15.18	(94)	6.18	28.9
evening	22.14	(108)				
night	22.59	(109)				
weekend, day	23.23	(107)				
Critical care, day	24.63	(82)				
OR, day	23.80	(41)				
ER, day	23.96	(48)				
Hospital nursing assistant:						
day	15.48	(99)	7.98	(84)	7.50	48.4
Nursing home RN services:						
day	24.21	(94)	16.07	(87)	8.14	33.6
evening	24.96	(94)	16.53	(85)	8.43	33.8
night	25.64	(93)	16.94	(84)	8.70	33.9
weekend, day	26.13	(93)	17.12	(83)	9.01	34.5
holiday, day	32.24	(77)	22.10	(79)	10.14	31.5
Nursing home LPN services:						
day	19.57	(94)	13.68	(95)	5.89	30.1
evening	20.24	(94)				
night	20.72	(94)				
weekend, day	21.31	(93)				
Nursing home CNA services:						
day	10.76	(95)	7.18	(96)	3.58	33.2
evening	11.04	(94)	7.29	(94)	3.75	34.0
night	11.26	(93)	7.34	(94)	3.92	34.8
weekend, day	11.66	(92)	7.54	(93)	4.12	35.3

39 reported providing 21.46% to nursing assistants. Of all the agencies, 45 indicated that their employees had a choice in selecting fringe benefits. In comparing registered nurses on per diem with salaried nurses and with contract nurses, the contract nurse was least likely to receive benefits. Per diem nurses were more likely to have workman's compensation, FICA, SUI, and FUI paid, while salaried nurses were more likely to receive paid benefits for vacation, sick leave, and health insurance, although less than 20% of agencies reported providing these benefits.

Liability insurance was another expense agencies reported. The quality of the information is limited, however, because some agencies reported this expense for an individual office and others for regional office, state office, or even their national expense level. Attempts to clarify this expense item during telephone interviews were not completely successful either because some respondents did not have the information or because the corporate office was unable to break down the expense for each local office. Of 84 agencies responding to the item about the annual cost of liability insurance, about three quarters indicated the premium was $500 to $15,000 annually. For others, premiums ranged up to $52,000. Several corporate offices indicated that the insurance premium for the firm ranged from $100,000 to $400,000 annually. One firm paid $0.88 per $100 of payroll. There were many levels of coverage ranging from $100,000 to $10 million per occurrence; however, most agencies indicated their coverage for liability was at $1 million per occurrence up to $3 million annually. Of the agencies responding, 84% indicated their policy covered personnel sent into the home, and 91% indicated that nurses assigned to the hospital setting were covered by the agency liability policy.

Many agencies did not report their charges, revenues, and expenses. Of the 54 agencies that reported both revenues and expenses, the average revenue for each firm was $1,612,661 and average expense per agency was $1,310,105. This is an excess of 18.8% of revenues over expenses. These figures hold little meaning, however, because it is not clear that they only represent revenue and expenses of the health personnel staffing services of a local office of a temporary staffing agency. It is likely that some reporting may have been done for an entire corporation or for subsidiaries within the firm other than health care supplemental staffing.

Conclusions

This study has described the use and costs of supplemental staffing agency personnel in Florida. Hospitals and nursing homes need to carefully review the reasons for using SSA personnel. The literature indicates that supplemental staffing may provide efficiency in labor costs for institutions having wide fluctuations in patient census and provide a "market answer" to the intrinsic sluggishness of nursing wages due to the monopsonistic character of the hospital and nursing home industry. Nursing homes with a stable census, however, may use supplemental staffing to fill vacant positions due to a shortage of personnel and temporary vacancies due to absences of regular staff.

The current study and studies cited in the literature provide a description of reasons that nurses select employment with temporary staffing agencies and give clear direction for corrections for hospitals and nursing homes that want to make less use of supplemental nurses from temporary staffing agencies. Hospitals and nursing homes should alter personnel policies to provide incentives for maintaining adequate staffing with their permanent staff or through in-house staffing pools.

Most agencies in this study did use written contacts with their institutional clients before placing nursing staff, and three quarters did this "only sometimes." The content of contracts varied among agencies. Such contractual agreements, in writing, may help to minimize some of the concerns voiced by the hospital and nursing home industries about SSAs. Contracts should address, at a minimum, issues related to qualifications and preemployment screening of personnel to be placed in the client's setting; the nature of orientation, supervision, and periodic evaluation of temporary staff; liability insurance requirements; scheduling and cancellation policies; charges; and other items of concern to either party. While JCAHO accreditation standards require such contracts, licensing or regulatory bodies for nursing homes do not. Depending on the situation, staffing services in individual patients' homes may not require such contracts.

The study of supplemental staffing agencies raises concerns for nursing practice and nursing personnel. The nurse who provides supplemental staffing often lacks the support of other staff colleagues and membership in a health team. The staffing nurse is usu-

ally considered to be an outsider who fills in and may be given undesirable tasks or may even experience resentment from the regular
staff at the placement site because of his or her salary and scheduling advantages. On the positive side, assignments in the patient's
home may provide opportunities for autonomy and independent
practice. Shifts in assignments provide a variety of experiences for
the nurse but may result in a lack of continuity in staffing and nursing care for the patient who is the recipient of services from different nurses. Shifts in assignment may make the staffing nurse more
vulnerable to making errors in administering medications or in
other aspects of care. This lack of institutional support has implications for nurses who may want to seek other sources of support,
such as in the professional association or by mechanisms built in by
the staffing agency to instill a sense of belonging in the agency
staff. This is particularly important for the inexperienced nurse.

Agencies deal with many issues when working with the staffing
nurse. Most nurses consider agency work short-term employment,
thus agencies must continually recruit new staff, which contributes
to turnover and mobility within the nursing profession. High mobility makes it easier for the unacceptable nurse to move from
agency to health setting for employment without being detected.
High turnover increases agency overhead costs for prescreening
and orienting employees. This, along with the variety of placement
settings, may contribute to the relatively short orientation and to
the evaluation and supervision problems related in this study. Although agency nurses have a wide latitude in scheduling options,
agencies must deal with absences by the nurse as well as late cancellations for staff by their hospital and nursing home clients. Responsibility for the nurses' actions is an area that is often unclear.
Unless contracts specify this clearly, liability for the staffing nurse's
actions may cause disputes between the agency and the hospital or
nursing home client. Liability for on-the-job injury raises similar issues and is another area that should be clarified in the agency-client
contract.

Some states have provided public policy responses to the growth
of temporary staffing through regulation of the industry. Such
trends raise the dilemma of whether increased regulation versus the
promotion of competition in the health care industry should occur.
At one extreme, states such as Massachusetts have passed legislation setting the rates charged by such agencies. Florida legislation

provides for passive registration of such agencies without further regulatory constraints.

Hospitals and nursing homes need to carefully review their reasons for using supplemental staffing agency personnel and the impact on costs and quality of care. Clearly, the emergence of supplemental staffing services in the mid-1970s with additional expansion since 1985 indicates that SSAs are a market response to greater forces in the health care industries. Policy responses directed solely to the temporary staffing agency will only postpone the work that needs to be done to reform the total health care system in the United States.

TEN

Recruitment and Retention of Nursing Personnel

WINIFRED H. SCHMELING

The importance to the health care industry of an adequate supply of professional nurses can hardly be overemphasized. During the past several years, nurse recruitment and retention have received increasing attention in the professional literature.

The conventional definition of *recruitment* has been to attract nurses to a particular place/position, while the definition of *retention* has been to keep them there. Recruitment and retention, however, are not so different. Recruitment is attracting people who are not on your staff yet. On the other hand, retention is recruiting your own staff every day!

There have been a variety of approaches to studying nurse recruitment and retention. One common approach has been to survey nurses to learn what they want (Huey & Hartley, 1988). Another approach has been to build complex mathematical models to explain turnover in terms of a number of demographic and organizational variables (Price & Mueller, 1981). Finally, the landmark Magnet Hospital Study used the approach of identifying exemplars to study what they do to attract and keep professional nurses (McClure et al., 1983).

This study included a large-scale data collection effort. Because the study was legislatively mandated and conducted under the data gathering authority of the Health Care Cost Containment Board, the response rate was virtually 100% of all hospitals, nursing homes, and home health agencies in the state. The data were collected in spring 1989.

The Florida legislature required that the study address the extent, causes, and impact of the nursing shortage. Early in the study, an extensive list of recruitment and retention strategies prominently mentioned in the literature during the last five years was generated. In an effort to understand what was being done in Florida to address the nursing shortage, and with what results, all respondents were asked to indicate whether they had never used the recruitment and/or recruitment and retention strategy listed. Respondents were also asked to rate the effectiveness of the strategy on a five-point scale. This resulted in an unusual picture of which strategies were being used in Florida and how the various affected industries rated the effectiveness of each strategy.

This chapter will summarize significant directions in the nurse recruitment and retention literature. In addition, the recruitment and retention findings from the study will be presented. Specific nurse recruitment and retention strategies used in Florida hospitals, nursing homes, and home health agencies, as well as industry ratings of their effectiveness, will be discussed. Finally, considerations will be raised regarding the fit between strategies suggested in the literature and those that have apparently been implemented in the various industry settings in Florida.

What We Know About Nurse Recruitment and Retention

Although there is understandably a great deal of interest in the health care industry in how to attract nurses to a particular institution, that is not our interest here. Many institution-specific, short-run strategies probably only succeed in producing internal movement in the marketplace. They do not really increase the supply of nurses. Our interest here is in examining what we know about nurse recruitment in the sense of increasing the number of nurses in the market.

The study examined the issue of increasing the supply of professional nurses and determined that, in general, the best recruitment strategies for increasing supply are those that influence the image of nursing and the career choices of young people.

During the past 20 years, there have been dramatic shifts in the career preferences of students entering college, particularly women students (Astin, Green, & Korn, 1987). Women's preferences are now more like men's preferences, shifting away from health and human services toward business, law, engineering, and medicine. Among male and female students, there is greater interest in material and power goals, coupled with decreased social concern and altruism. The image of nursing has never fit with material and power goals. It is increasingly not seen as a viable choice for the best and brightest—certainly not for men and, more recently, not for women either.

Image is very important in career choice. Occupational image is a generalization made about a particular occupation, including the personalities of people in those jobs, the type of work they do, the type of lives they lead, the rewards and conditions of work, and the appropriateness of the job for different types of people. Occupational images include sex types and prestige levels. Career choice is a developmental process. Sex type impressions are formed between the ages of 6 and 8; prestige-level impressions are formed between the ages of 9 and 13; and unique preferences are established beginning around the age of 14 (Gottfredson, 1981).

For these reasons, the best recruitment strategies probably involve enhancing the image of nursing and working to influence career choice among school-age children. Such strategies would include educational outreach, career counseling, career days, open houses for students, and so on.

In general, the most promising short-run strategies for actually increasing supply involve affiliating with schools of nursing to attract graduating students. Although nursing school enrollments have recently increased, this is not expected to be a long-term trend. Most of the increase has been accounted for by dipping into the pool of nontraditional students, particularly more mature women (Roberts, Minnick, Ginsberg, & Curran, 1989).

Because the current nursing shortage is characterized by fewer people entering nursing and by the relative lack of unemployed nurses, maintaining an adequate supply of nurses must include a focus on preventing vacancies. Not only is turnover expensive, it can also negatively affect job satisfaction, which further affects turnover.

Nursing retention has also been studied a great deal. The most definitive recent work has been done by the Hospital Research and Education Trust (Curran & Minnick, 1989). They had intended to conduct a large-scale data collection effort to build a mathematical model that would identify those factors that account for turnover. To their surprise, they learned that the influencing factors are numerous and their relationships vary with demographics and from institution to institution.

Their findings (Curran & Minnick, 1989) are summarized in three principles:

Principle 1. Retention is affected by the interaction of multiple internal and external factors, which are difficult to predict universally due to the complexity of their interrelationships.

Principle 2. Each institution must develop retrievable data gathered during an ongoing organizational assessment.

Principle 3. Strategies and tactics to improve retention must be highly individualized by matching findings from the ongoing assessment to identified demands.

This work suggests that the best nurse retention strategies are specific to the institution and are based on a periodic survey of the nursing staff. These retention strategies are based on specific demographic and preference data and are developed with extensive staff involvement.

Recruitment and Retention Findings

All hospital, nursing home, and home health agency respondents to the study questionnaire were asked to give their opinions on the effectiveness of various recruitment and retention strategies. The strategies listed were generated during the literature review for the study.

STRATEGIES

The first group were primarily recruitment strategies. The second group were primarily retention strategies, but many overlapped. Respondents were asked to indicate with a check those strategies they had never used and to rate their impression of the effectiveness of the strategies on a five-point scale, with 1 meaning not effective and 5, very effective. Definitions were provided with the instructions. Respondents were permitted to rate the effectiveness of the strategy even if they had never personally used it. Response rates varied. In general, respondents who had used the strategy were more likely to rate it.

TABLE 10.1 Recruitment Strategies for Hospitals

Strategy	Percentage Never Used	Percentage Rating 1 or 2	Percentage Rating 4 or 5
Nurse recruitment centers	74.81	67.65	7.35
Career counseling:			
junior high school	51.66	44.27	25.95
senior high school	37.69	39.66	28.49
junior college	35.74	39.13	32.07
college	37.79	40.23	29.31
Local educational outreach	56.32	42.75	19.08
Job placement programs	62.87	57.43	13.86
Out-of-state recruitment	28.78	53.00	14.50
Foreign nurse recruitment	57.14	56.15	15.38
Career days	18.15	50.43	18.70
Direct mail advertising	46.01	51.68	23.49
Newspaper advertising	2.15	27.68	36.53
Radio/TV advertising	72.10	51.55	16.49
Convention booths	34.53	69.23	9.34
Job fairs	22.74	67.29	11.68
Open house for students	38.63	40.59	31.18
Programs for counselors	64.03	42.00	22.00
Affiliation with nursing schools	17.82	14.16	62.39

NOTE: A rating of 1-2 indicates ineffective; a rating of 4-5 indicates effective.

Hospitals. Table 10.1 shows the percentage of hospitals that reported they had never used the recruitment and/or retention strategy. Because Florida had no nurse recruitment center at the time of the survey, it is not surprising that three fourths of the hospitals reported never using a strategy. A majority, however, did not have programs for school counselors, job placement programs, local educational outreach, or career counseling at the junior high school level. A surprising 38% never had open houses for students. Career counseling was not done at any level by 35%-37% of the hospitals. Recruitment efforts were focused on newspaper advertising, affiliation with nursing schools, career days, and job fairs.

Apparently, 85% of the hospitals have no programs in place to help employees cope with the stress of balancing work and other life demands. Nearly three fourths have not tried innovative practice models such as case management or shared governance and are not involved in research. Nearly two thirds have not instituted any work redesign.

TABLE 10.2 Recruitment and Retention Strategies for Hospitals

Strategy	Percentage Never Used	Percentage Rating 1 or 2	Percentage Rating 4 or 5
Increased salaries	2.14	10.62	64.84
Increased salary ranges	3.93	9.92	67.18
Child-care programs	53.21	19.85	53.44
Innovative benefit structures	23.74	14.49	56.04
Nursing image enhancement	23.30	21.03	49.53
Internships	44.09	18.59	48.08
Preceptorships	7.17	19.71	57.69
Tuition reimbursement	7.58	20.00	51.76
In-house registry	33.70	20.22	51.91
Weekend program	33.69	15.14	59.46
Part-time flexibility	7.12	16.09	61.30
10- to 12-hour shifts	12.54	13.52	63.52
4- to 6-hour shifts	49.10	31.69	40.14
Clinical career ladders	52.90	23.08	42.31
In-service education programs	3.93	25.47	38.20
Job satisfaction surveys	28.62	44.67	18.27
Paid conference time	17.50	30.74	35.93
Mentoring	44.77	30.72	39.22
Career counseling	52.77	37.50	20.31
Living with work programs	84.50	47.73	22.73
Involvement in research	72.83	51.19	25.00
Computer training	56.25	59.17	12.50
Alternative models of practice:			
case management	75.09	33.85	35.38
shared governance	74.73	27.54	44.93
work redesign	64.66	21.28	43.62

NOTE: A rating of 1-2 indicates ineffective; a rating of 4-5 indicates effective.

And more than half have not offered computer training, child care, or clinical career ladders or career counseling. The most widely used strategies were increasing salary and salary ranges and offering in-service education, part-time flexibility, preceptorships, tuition reimbursement, 10- to 12-hour shifts, and paid conference time. About three fourths of the hospitals have conducted job satisfaction surveys that could serve as the basis for institution-specific retention programs (Table 10.2).

Nursing homes. Nursing homes were less likely to have used any of the listed recruitment strategies (Table 10.3). Least used were

TABLE 10.3 Recruitment Strategies for Nursing Homes

Strategy	Percentage Never Used	Percentage Rating 1 or 2	Percentage Rating 4 or 5
Nurse recruitment centers	83.15	70.67	8.00
Career counseling:			
junior high school	72.35	68.33	10.83
senior high school	60.75	62.80	17.07
junior college	57.04	58.06	15.59
college	63.53	60.65	16.77
Local educational outreach	54.61	59.70	13.93
Job placement programs	33.48	57.77	14.19
Out-of-state recruitment	78.89	74.74	10.53
Foreign nurse recruitment	76.99	57.69	25.96
Career days	53.56	71.77	6.22
Direct mail advertising	73.44	53.78	14.29
Newspaper advertising	7.96	19.71	37.50
Radio/TV advertising	79.73	63.74	10.99
Convention booths	67.92	75.86	7.59
Job fairs	63.25	72.12	9.09
Open house for students	69.84	58.09	15.44
Programs for counselors	83.41	52.70	14.86
Affiliation with nursing schools	46.36	39.83	34.75

NOTE: a rating of 1-2 indicates ineffective; a rating of 4-5 indicates effective.

programs for school counselors. Well over half never used career counseling at any level, educational outreach, open houses for students, or career days. Nearly half did not affiliate with nursing schools. The most widely used recruitment strategy was newspaper ads.

Most nursing homes have not implemented recruitment and retention strategies beyond raising salaries, offering in-service education, tuition reimbursement, and part-time flexibility(Table 10.4). More than 90% have not tried living with work programs or involvement in research. Over 80% have no preceptorships, internships, or child care programs and are not involved in work redesign or innovative practice models. About three fourths to two thirds do not offer mentoring, career counseling, clinical career ladders, or flexible shifts. Nearly half have not done job satisfaction surveys.

Home health agencies. Home health agencies are even less likely than nursing homes to use the recruitment strategies recognized in

TABLE 10.4 Recruitment and Retention Strategies for Nursing Homes

Strategy	Percentage Never Used	Percentage Rating 1 or 2	Percentage Rating 4 or 5
Increased salaries	3.08	12.73	57.05
Increased salary ranges	14.63	14.81	54.55
Child-care programs	83.81	24.66	46.58
Innovative benefit structures	38.08	28.42	43.53
Nursing image enhancement	46.40	38.24	30.67
Internships	82.29	41.77	29.11
Preceptorships	81.12	39.29	28.57
Tuition reimbursement	32.89	42.00	28.33
In-house registry	74.33	39.13	33.04
Weekend program	61.74	23.39	46.20
Part-time flexibility	21.25	33.24	38.64
10- to 12-hour shifts	55.80	36.87	39.39
4- to 6-hour shifts	67.34	47.59	22.76
Clinical career ladders	64.21	44.38	26.88
In-service education programs	11.83	49.37	20.76
Job satisfaction surveys	48.76	53.95	21.93
Paid conference time	30.96	45.81	22.90
Mentoring	73.26	51.52	34.34
Career counseling	68.90	48.20	15.83
Living with work programs	91.82	52.78	13.89
Involvement in research	90.42	69.77	11.63
Computer training	88.99	45.90	18.03
Alternative models of practice:			
case management	85.34	45.90	18.03
shared governance	87.25	46.15	30.77
work redesign	83.70	38.24	33.82

NOTE: A rating of 1-2 indicates ineffective; a rating of 4-5 indicates effective.

the literature (Table 10.5). Nearly half did nothing except advertise in the newspapers. Very few have implemented strategies that would increase supply. Most do not affiliate with nursing schools or participate in job fairs or career days.

Home health agencies are much more likely to implement innovative practice models such as case management. Only 28% have never used this strategy, compared with about 85% of the nursing homes and 75% of the hospitals. They are also more likely to offer living with work programs and career counseling. Three fourths, however, offer no shared governance or computer training. Two

TABLE 10.5 Recruitment Strategies for Home Health Agencies

Strategy	Percentage Never Used	Percentage Rating 1 or 2	Percentage Rating 4 or 5
Nurse recruitment centers	64.68	61.90	0.00
Career counseling:			
junior high school	81.03	67.65	17.65
senior high school	74.73	46.51	18.60
junior college	63.74	43.94	18.18
college	59.12	52.70	18.92
Local educational outreach	61.81	51.52	21.21
Job placement programs	55.94	66.29	8.99
Out-of-state recruitment	74.63	64.71	17.65
Foreign nurse recruitment	56.52	72.73	9.09
Career days	47.03	49.11	10.71
Direct mail advertising	57.56	54.55	19.32
Newspaper advertising	2.44	10.91	55.76
Radio/TV advertising	77.83	57.78	17.78
Convention booths	46.77	57.94	12.15
Job fairs	49.76	57.14	8.79
Open house for students	70.73	56.14	10.53
Programs for counselors	84.88	45.16	19.35
Affiliation with nursing schools	58.67	38.27	30.86

NOTE: A rating of 1-2 indicates ineffective; a rating of 4-5 indicates effective.

thirds offer no preceptorships, internships, child-care programs, mentoring, or work redesign. And about 40% have not done job satisfaction surveys. The most commonly used recruitment and retention strategies are increased salaries, clinical career ladders, part-time flexibility, nursing image enhancement, and in-service education programs (Table 10.6).

STRATEGIES RATED INEFFECTIVE

The respondents rated the effectiveness of various recruitment and retention strategies. Strategies rated 1 or 2 on the five-point scale are reported here as ineffective.

Hospitals. More than half of the hospitals rated the following as ineffective recruitment strategies: convention booths, nurse recruitment centers, job fairs, foreign nurse recruitment, out-of-state recruit-

TABLE 10.6 Recruitment and Retention Strategies for Home Health Agencies

Strategy	Percentage Never Used	Percentage Rating 1 or 2	Percentage Rating 4 or 5
Increased salaries	8.25	9.63	65.24
Increased salary ranges	15.69	11.63	63.95
Child-care programs	66.18	20.00	46.15
Innovative benefit structures	33.82	32.86	44.29
Nursing image enhancement	15.76	32.62	36.88
Internships	70.79	47.46	28.81
Preceptorships	66.34	36.49	32.43
Tuition reimbursement	43.41	34.48	37.93
Part-time flexibility	15.20	10.40	63.01
Clinical career ladders	12.32	20.00	30.00
In-service education programs	16.02	37.57	31.79
Job satisfaction surveys	39.41	50.41	17.89
Paid conference time	26.37	34.81	31.65
Mentoring	61.00	43.59	26.92
Career counseling	6.93	59.02	18.03
Living with work programs	4.68	57.69	11.54
Involvement in research	58.91	60.61	21.21
Computer training	78.50	51.16	13.95
Alternative models of practice:			
case management	28.21	25.36	50.72
shared governance	71.74	38.46	38.46
work redesign	63.04	32.35	35.29

NOTE: A rating of 1-2 indicates ineffective; a rating of 4-5 indicates effective.

ment, direct mail advertising, radio/TV advertising, and career days. It is surprising that more than 40% rated as ineffective career counseling and open houses for school students, educational outreach, and programs for school counselors. Their lowest rating was for affiliation with nursing schools.

Fewer hospitals rated recruitment and retention strategies as ineffective, although more than half rated computer training and involvement in research as ineffective. Almost half rated living with work programs and job satisfaction surveys as ineffective. Their lowest ratings were for increasing salaries and salary ranges and offering 10- to 12-hour shifts, innovative benefit structures, weekend programs, part-time flexibility, preceptorships, and internships.

Nursing homes. Nursing homes were more likely to rate recruit-ment and retention strategies ineffective. More than half rated virtu-ally all of the strategies ineffective, with the exception of affiliation with nursing schools (40%) and newspaper advertising (20%).

Many nursing homes see as ineffective strategies that have been in the literature for some time. They rate them as ineffective in many cases even though they have never tried them. More than half rated the following ineffective: involvement in research, job satisfaction surveys, living with work programs, and mentoring. Nearly half rated as ineffective in-service education programs, career counsel-ing, 4- to 6-hour shifts, shared governance, computer training, case management, paid conference time, and clinical career ladders. The lowest ratings were for increasing salaries.

Home health agencies. Home health agencies also gave relatively low ratings to most of the recruitment strategies. The strategies they considered most ineffective were foreign nurse recruitment, career counseling at the junior high level, job placement programs, and out-of-state recruitment. Their lowest ratings were for newspaper advertising and affiliation with nursing schools.

More than half of the home health agencies rated the following as ineffective recruitment and retention strategies: involvement in re-search, career counseling, living with work programs, computer training, and job satisfaction surveys. Nearly half also thought mentoring and internships were ineffective strategies. They gave their lowest ratings to increased salaries and part-time flexibility.

STRATEGIES RATED EFFECTIVE

The respondents rated the effectiveness of various recruitment and retention strategies. Strategies rated 4 or 5 on the five-point scale are reported as effective.

Hospitals. More than 60% of the hospitals surveyed rated affiliat-ing with schools of nursing as an effective recruitment strategy. The next highest ratings, at about one third, were for newspaper adver-tising, career counseling at the junior college level, and open houses for students.

Hospitals rate increased salary ranges (67%) and salaries (64%) followed by 10- to 12-hour shifts (63%) and part-time flexibility (61%) as the most effective recruitment and retention strategies. A number of strategies that have been in the literature for some time were rated effective by less than half of the hospitals; for example, nursing image enhancement, mentoring, internships, shared governance, work redesign, and clinical career ladders. Less than 20% considered job satisfaction surveys an effective strategy.

Nursing homes. Most nursing home respondents did not see any of the recruitment strategies as very effective. The highest effectiveness ratings were for newspaper advertising (37%) and affiliation with nursing schools (34%). The lowest ratings were for career days, convention booths, nurse recruitment centers, and job fairs.

Only two recruitment and retention strategies are rated as effective by more than half of the nursing home respondents: increased salaries (57%) and increased salary ranges (54%). Only 21% rated job satisfaction surveys as effective. Their lowest rating was for involvement in research.

Home health agencies. Only one recruitment strategy was rated as effective by the home health agency respondents—newspaper advertising (55%). The next highest rating was for affiliation with nursing schools (30%). The remaining strategies were rated effective by less than 20% of the respondents. The lowest ratings were for nurse recruitment centers, job fairs, job placement programs, foreign nurse recruitment, and open houses for students.

Four recruitment and retention strategies were rated as effective by more than half the home health agency respondents: increased salaries and salary ranges, part-time flexibility, and the case management practice model. The strategies rated as effective by the fewest respondents were living with work programs, computer training, and job satisfaction surveys (17%).

Conclusions: Are the Myths Alive and Well?

In general, there is not a particularly good fit between what has been recommended in the literature for a number of years and the nurse recruitment and retention strategies being implemented in Florida's health care industry. Of the three types of health care organizations, hospitals fit the directions somewhat more closely.

NURSE RECRUITMENT

The most commonly used nurse recruitment and retention strategies are increasing salaries and salary ranges and advertising in newspapers. These strategies are consistent with belief in the myth that nurses are "out there" and it is just a question of telling them you are interested and making it lucrative enough to attract them. To the degree that these strategies are effective, they do not really increase the actual supply of nurses.

Most hospitals affiliate with schools of nursing, but, even when they do, they are not as likely to hold open houses for students. And most facilities have little interest in working with public schools to increase the number of students selecting nursing as a career.

NURSE RETENTION

Again, increasing salary and salary ranges is seen as the most effective nurse retention strategy and is the most frequently used. Most facilities have little interest in, nor do they see as effective, strategies that are prevalent in the literature such as innovative practice models and work redesign. The exception is the home health industry, which uses the case management model.

Hospitals were far more likely to use job satisfaction surveys (28% never used) than home health agencies (39% never used) or nursing homes (48% never used). It is not clear how they were using the data generated by these surveys. None of the three types of organizations was particularly excited about the effectiveness of job satisfaction surveys in nurse retention. The percentage rating it effective was hospitals (18%), nursing homes (21%), and home health agencies (17%).

None of the organizations showed an interest in developing and providing programs to assist nurses in dealing with the stress of work or balancing work and other life priorities. And there was little interest in involvement with research or working with nursing staff to develop career goals.

Work redesign, widely regarded as an absolute necessity to relieve the nurse of nonnursing duties, was never used by 64% of the hospitals, 63% of the home health agencies, and 83% of the nursing homes. It was seen as an effective strategy by only 43% of the hospitals, 35% of the home health agencies, and 33% of the nursing homes.

In summary, there is not a good fit between the nurse recruitment and retention strategies recommended in the literature and those in current use. Furthermore, organizations seem to have determined that strategies are not effective without having ever tried them. The strategies rated most effective in all three types of organizations are newspaper advertising and increasing salaries and salary ranges.

ELEVEN

The Competitive Employment Market for Nurses

WILLIAM J. SEROW

MARIE E. COWART

In the last two decades, the health system has shifted from largely public and not-for-profit ownership to considerable proprietary involvement. The industry shifted from a period of unbridled expansion in the 1950s and early 1960s, to a period of concern for equity in the late 1960s and early 1970s, to a period late in the 1970s through the current time when cost containment is the prime interest. Alternative delivery systems emphasizing ambulatory and community-based services expanded as an alternative to high-cost institutional care. As services changed, the demand for nurses increased and alternative labor markets for nurses expanded. By the time of our study, not only had competition for nursing personnel increased but employment practices in settings hiring nurses had undergone change because of increased technology, prospective hospital reimbursement, and increased specialization. Thus the emphasis in this study of institutions and agencies in several health industries provides a fresh perspective on the study of nursing personnel.

This chapter is designed to integrate the findings from the several chapters that deal with issues pertaining to the employment of nurses in the specific industries that jointly constitute the health care sector. The primary intent of this chapter is not merely to summarize or recapitulate the results presented in those chapters but is an effort to encompass them into an integrated portrait of the labor market for nurses as it exists in Florida. In general, the approach to be taken here is to compare and contrast among employers of nurses—hospitals, nursing homes, community settings (that is, home health agencies, hospices, and public health agencies), and temporary or supplemental staffing agencies. We begin with a description of the employers themselves, based on their size, ownership, and location within Florida. This is followed by a profile of the nursing staff within each of these types of facilities, including the mixture of types of nursing personnel and characteristics of personnel, including age, length of service, and level of education. The third section focuses upon the relative degree and severity of shortage and turnover and also incorporates comparative information on factors contributing to shortages, including salary and benefit levels. The fourth section compares the responses of the various types of institutions to the shortage, including service alternations; additional expense for overtime, temporary staff, and recruiting; and changes in staff mix and substitution strategies. This section concludes with a summary of the use and perceived effectiveness of alternative recruitment and retention strategies.

Comparative Characteristics of Employing Institutions

Tables 11.1 to 11.4 illustrate some of the more salient characteristics of those institutions that provide the vast majority of employment opportunities for nursing personnel. In terms of ownership, an overwhelming majority of both nursing homes and temporary staffing agencies indicated that they were proprietary, that is, for-profit institutions. Almost two thirds of home health agencies and very nearly half of all hospitals also reported this form of ownership. All of the 29 hospices included in the sample were private, not-for-profit entities. Only among hospitals, then, could it be said that there exists much in the way of diversity in terms of ownership of institutions. The overall mix of institutions is represented by a higher proportion with proprietary ownership than in the national averages. For example, the 45% of Florida hospitals with this form of ownership is nearly four times the national proportion. Similarly, the 87% of proprietarily operated nursing homes exceeds the national average by some 12 percentage points (Harrington, 1991).

In terms of their geographic distribution across Florida, Table 11.2 groups the institutions into a tripartite division of north, central,

TABLE 11.1 Ownership of Employing Institutions

Measure Ownership	Hospitals		Nursing Homes		Home Health Agencies		Hospices		Temporary Staffing Agencies	
	N	%	N	%	N	%	N	%	N	%
Public	42	15	8	2	8	4	0	0	0	0
Not for profit	108	38	49	11	69	33	29	100	10	5
For Profit	132	47	401	87	134	63	0	0	175*	95
Total	282	100	458	100	211	100	29	100	185	100

*Includes 6 for profit subsidiaries of not-for-profit hospitals; a total of 12 agencies are owned by hospitals or hospital groups and 4 are owned by nursing homes or nursing home groups.

and south Florida. A disproportionately large number of both hospitals and nursing homes are located in the northern portion of the state, while a disproportionately small number of both are located in the south. This in and of itself is *not* an indication of a maldistribution of health care resources, because most of the state's smaller facilities are in northern Florida and many of the largest are located in south Florida. Disproportionately large numbers of both nursing homes and temporary staffing agencies are to be found in central Florida, largely reflecting the distribution of the state's elderly population.

Direct comparisons among the employers with respect to their size are quite difficult to draw, given the nature of their missions. One might observe that, while the mean size of hospitals is some 224 beds, nearly 60% of these facilities have fewer than 200 beds, suggesting a somewhat skewed distribution. Regulations control-

TABLE 11.2 Location of Employing Institutions

Location	Hospitals		Nursing Homes		Home Health Agencies		Hospices		Temporary Staffing Agencies*		Florida Population %
	N	%	N	%	N	%	N	%	N	%	%
North	91	32	138	30	46	22	9	31	26	15	25
Central	84	29	160	35	65	31	8	28	69	39	28
South	110	39	161	35	100	47	12	41	81	46	46
Total	285	100	459	100	211	100	29	100	176	100	100

*Excludes 21 out-of-state agencies.

TABLE 11.3 Size of Employing Institutions

Size (number of beds)	Hospitals N	%	Size (number of beds or average daily census) (NH)	(HHA/Hos)	Nursing Homes N	%	Home Health Agencies N	%	Hospices N	%
0-99	66	27	0-59	1-49	42	9	94	49	11	38
100-199	76	31	60-89	50-99	70	15	41	21	13	45
200-299	39	16	90-119	100-149	67	15	23	12	1	3
300-399	23	9	120-149	150+	184	40	33	17	4	14
400-499	13	5	150-179		31	7				
500+	29	12	180+		65	14				
Total	246	100			459	100	191	100	29	100
Mean	224				120		85		82	

ling the allocation of nursing home beds are such that many of these facilities have exactly 120 beds; this is reflected in the bed-size distribution of nursing homes, with fully 40% of them being in the 120-149 bed category.

Table 11.4 presents the average number of nurses, by level of preparation, employed in each setting. While the measures available for this are not constant across types, it is possible to draw some general conclusions. First, given the difference in mission, it is hardly surprising that hospitals employ more than three times the number of nurses per occupied bed than do nursing homes. Second, and also reflective of differing goals, is the difference in the distribution of employed nurses according to their level of preparation. About two thirds of nurses employed in the average hospital are registered nurses (RNs), in contrast to about 15% of those nurses

TABLE 11.4 Number of Nurses Employed in Institutions

Number of Employed Nurses*	Hospitals	Nursing Homes	Home Health Agencies	Hospices	Temporary Staffing Agencies
RNs	102.5	6.4	0.24	NA	51
LPNs	30.8	10.9	0.4	NA	97
NAs	32.9	34.8	0.37	NA	74
Total	166.2	52.1	1.01	NA	222

*Number of full-time equivalent per 100 occupied beds for hospitals and nursing homes; FTE ratio to average daily census for HHAs; average number of employees for TSAs.

employed by nursing homes and a fourth of those in hospices. The staff of the average nursing home was heavily concentrated in nursing assistants (NAs—about two thirds of the staff), while these nurses and licensed practical nurses (LPNs) each constituted some 40% of the staff of the average hospice. Finally, nearly half of the average roster of temporary staffing agencies is made up of LPNs, with about a fourth RNs and about a third NAs; these would presumably reflect the demand of the agency's clients for specific types of nursing personnel.

Nationally, in 1987 the same proportions of the various levels of personnel are found, on average, in hospitals (*Seventh Report to the President and Congress*, 1990). The proportion of nursing assistants in nursing homes for the entire nation was 71%, somewhat higher than the level observed in Florida, but, in home health agencies, the share of this category of personnel was similar in that of the state and the nation. The relative mix of registered nurses to licensed practical nurses and nursing assistants has implications for the role of the nurse in the respective settings. Contrasting hospitals (where the registered nurse spends an average of 45 minutes per day per patient) to nursing homes (6 to 12 minutes per patient per day) indicates that more time is spent in the latter on directing and supervising rather than on providing direct care (Harrington, 1991). Yet the hiring practices in nursing homes, where high proportions of diploma- and associate degree-prepared nurses, rather than geriatric nurse practitioners, are employed, indicates that the nature of skills needed for the respective settings is not taken into account when hiring.

Characteristics of Nurses
Employed in Different Settings

Table 11.5 presents data that depict some of the characteristics of those nurses who are employed in each of the particular settings. The most striking finding in terms of the age structure of the nursing staff is the considerable disparity between those employed in nursing homes and those employed in all other settings. The median age of the former, 49 years, is more than 10 years greater than that for all nursing personnel and is fully 7 years more than the median age in the next highest category (hospices, at 42 years). The overall age distribution of those nurses employed by temporary staffing agencies is strikingly different than that found in other settings,

TABLE 11.5 Summary Characteristics of Professional Nurses, by Type
of Employing Institution, 1988

Percentage Distribution	*Hospitals*	*Nursing Homes*	*Home Health Agencies*	*Hospices*	*Temporary Staffing Agencies*
Age for RNs:					
under 25	3	1	3	1	12
25-34	30	14	32	20	31
35-44	34	24	35	41	26
45-54	21	29	21	24	12
55-64	10	23	8	15	7
65 and over	2	9	1	0	11
median	40	49	39	42	38
Length of employment:*					
< 1 year	27	33	44	42	29
1-5 years	35	44	45	41	35
6-10 years	21	20	9	4	16
11-20 years	13	2	3	0	9
> 20 years	5	1	0	4	11
Median	3.5	2.5	1.5	1.8	3.4
Educational preparation for RNs:					
associate	51	33	48	60	41
diploma	28	44	29	25	28
baccalaureate	18	20	21	13	25
graduate	3	3	2	2	6

*RNs and LPNs for all but TSAs; only RNs for TSAs.

with a substantially greater portion at both ends of the age spectrum. This would suggest that this means of employment is especially attractive both to those just entering the profession as well as those most likely to be interested in part-time or occasional assignments. Thus agencies would seem to provide the youngest members of the profession an opportunity to "try out" employment in a variety of settings before making a more permanent commitment to one of them and, at the same time, afford nurses who wish to pursue their craft on a more sporadic basis an opportunity to do so.

Hospitals and temporary staffing agencies stand apart from other settings in terms of the longevity of their staff (middle panel of Table 11.5). The median duration of employment in these is about three and a half years, or some one to two years longer than elsewhere. As might be anticipated, these figures offer a clue to differences in vacancy and, especially, turnover rates among the different employment settings.

The final characteristic of professional nurses illustrated in Table 11.5 is the variation in their type of educational preparation across employment settings. These are shown in the third and final panel. The extent of this variation is not great and is perhaps largely reflective of those variations in age structure described above. These data, which apply only to registered nurses, show a much greater concentration of diploma-trained nurses in the nursing home setting than is true elsewhere. In Florida, the number of hospital-based diploma programs has been gradually reduced over time and now includes only a single representative. To a considerable extent, these have been superseded by associate degree programs offered through the community college system. While the relatively high percentage of nurses with diploma preparation could be attributed to the relative older age of the nursing home nurse, there were proportionately fewer nurses with this preparation in all industries in Florida than was true nationally. In 1988, the national average for preparation among registered nurses was 49% diploma, 28% associate degree, 22% baccalaureate, and 0.1% with graduate degrees (*Seventh Report to the President and Congress,* 1990).

Also of note in this regard is the larger proportion of nurses employed by temporary staffing agencies who possess one or more degrees from four-year institutions of higher education. This may reflect the relatively large number of the youngest nurses employed by this sector, or the temporary assignment sector may be the employment choice for nurses desiring part-time work while going to school.

Vacancy and Turnover Rates
in Alternative Employment Settings

Summary data on vacancy and turnover rates for professional nurses, arrayed according to level of nurse preparation and type and salient characteristics of employment setting, are given in Table 11.6. With respect first to vacancy rates (upper panel), the hospice sector is notable for possessing considerably lower vacancy rates (under 10% regardless of the level of preparation) than found elsewhere. In the other three settings for which data are available, vacancy rates are considerably higher than those observed for hospices, with

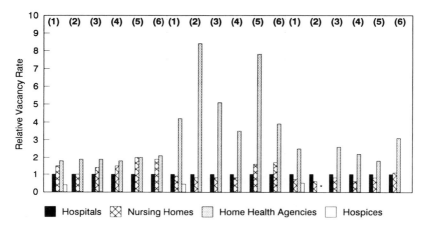

Figure 11.1. Relative Vacancy Rates Among Professional Nurses by Level of Preparation and Type of Employment Setting (hospitals = 1.0)
NOTE: 1 = total, 2 = public, 3 = nonprofit, 4 = proprietary, 5 = largest, and 6 = smallest.
*Not available.

home health agencies generally experiencing levels considerably in excess of those found in either hospitals or nursing homes. This is shown graphically in Figure 11.1, which expresses vacancy rates for each sector relative to those observed in hospitals.

There also exist fairly uniform patterns of variation in vacancy rates according to the size and mode of ownership of the employer. In terms of the size of the institution, the general tendency is that vacancy rates are inversely related to the size of the employing institution; this is clearly the case for each level of nurse preparation and across all three institutional types for which detailed data are available.

These differences are somewhat less clear-cut with respect to ownership. In the case of nursing homes, vacancy rates are at a minimum in publicly owned facilities and at a maximum for proprietaries, but it should be remembered that there exist only a handful of the former. For-profit hospitals usually have more problems with vacancies among their LPN and NA positions than do the two other ownership forms, but this is not the case for RNs, for whom there is little overall difference. Finally, there does not appear to be any systematic relationship between vacancy rates and ownership for home health agencies.

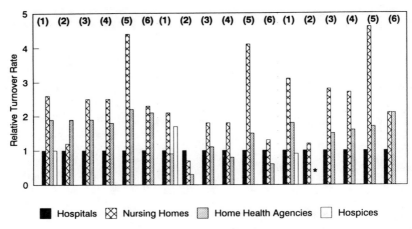

Figure 11.2. Relative Turnover Rates Among Professional Nurses by Level of Preparation and Type of Employment Setting (hospitals = 1.0)
NOTE: 1 = total, 2 = public, 3 = nonprofit, 4 = proprietary, 5 = largest, and 6 = smallest.

The lower panel of Table 11.6 provides data on turnover rates and, once again, the lowest levels are usually found in the hospice sector, although the margin of difference relative to other sectors is less here than in the case of vacancy rates and in fact is higher than that found in the public sector for the case of LPNs. Nursing homes tend to experience much higher levels of turnover than do other sectors, with differentials relative to hospitals of 100% or more not uncommon. These high rates reflect much about the nursing home setting. For the registered nurse and the licensed practical nurse, this sector might be considered a last alternative. In interviews, nursing home nurses reported they were stigmatized by their peers in hospital settings, who exhibited little understanding of the specialty skills and career satisfaction found in the nursing home setting (Speake, Cowart, & Schmeling, 1990). While the major employment competitor for RNs and LPNs is the hospital, for the nursing assistant (a position in which turnover is at a maximum), the hospitality industry also provides alternative job opportunities. Figure 11.2 expresses turnover rates for each sector relative to those observed in hospitals.

Again, as was the case for vacancy rates, there is a consistent and pronounced inverse relationship between size of the employing institution and level of turnover. There is also a more well-grounded and consistent differential with regard to the ownership of the particular entity; in most instances, it could be concluded that the progression from lowest to highest turnover follows the path from publicly owned to not for profit to proprietary.

To summarize these data, vacancy rates are much lower in hospices and much higher in home health agencies than is true in the other two settings for all levels of nurse preparation. Hospitals collectively experience less vacancy in their budgeted RN positions than do nursing homes, but this situation is reversed for NA positions. Hospices and hospitals usually experience lesser degrees of turnover than do home health agencies and, especially, nursing homes, where turnover is especially problematic.

Perceived Severity of the Shortage

In addition to the largely objective measures of shortage and turnover that respondents were asked to provide, the survey also afforded them the opportunity to indicate their own perceptions of the degree of severity of shortage that they faced in their own context. For purposes of comparison across components of the overall health care industry, Table 11.7 extracts these responses, showing the mean score reported by hospitals, nursing homes, hospices, and home health care agencies, with degree of severity scored on an ascending scale from 1 to 5. Furthermore, the degree of severity was posed according to season of the year, day of the week, and shift.

The responses to this inquiry were largely as one would expect and display only modest variation across sectors. The sectors are uniform in their assessments that (a) the fall and winter months represent the time of year when the shortage is most acute (reflecting the large volume of tourism and part-time residents in Florida; (b) weekends are more problematic than a representative (Wednesday) day in the middle of the week; and (c) shortage is much more of a problem on the evening and night shifts than on the day shift. As a general statement, it could be said fairly that hospices tended to view the situation with slightly less gravity than did the other sectors, a conclusion quite consistent with the comparatively modest vacancy rates for that sector shown in Table 11.6.

NURSES IN THE WORKPLACE

TABLE 11.6 Measures of Shortage of Professional Nurses, by Type of Employing Institution, 1988

Measure	Hospitals	Nursing Homes	Home Health Agencies	Hospices	Temporary Staffing Agencies
Vacancy rate:					
RNs—total	17	25	31	7	NA
public	19	19	37		
NFP	17	24	33		
proprietary	17	25	30		
largest	12	24	24		
smallest	19	37	40		
LPNs—total	20	18	83	9	NA
public	11	9	92		
NFP	17	13	86		
proprietary	24	19	83		
largest	19	14	70		
smallest	23	38	89		
NAs—total	18	12	45	9	NA
public	18	10	NA		
NFP	14	11	37		
proprietary	22	13	48		
largest	13	11	24		
smallest	19	21	59		
Turnover rate:					
RNs—total	28	74	52	28	NA
public	21	26	39		
NFP	26	66	49		
proprietary	31	76	55		
largest	18	79	39		
smallest	33	77	70		
LPNs—total	33	69	30	55	NA
public	24	16	8		
NFP	28	49	31		
proprietary	39	72	30		
largest	15	62	22		
smallest	47	61	93		
NAs—total	37	114	67	34	NA
public	32	37	NA		
NFP	31	86	46		
proprietary	44	118	72		
largest	21	96	35		
smallest	44	93	94		

TABLE 11.7 Industry Perceptions of the Seriousness of Nurses Shortage

Period	Hospitals	Nursing Homes	Home Health Agencies	Hospices
Season:				
spring	2.7	3.0	2.9	2.6
summer	2.3	3.1	2.7	2.3
fall	3.0	3.0	3.1	3.2
winter	3.5	3.1	3.5	3.1
Day of week:				
Wednesday	2.3	2.3	2.7	2.1
Saturday	3.6	3.8	3.8	3.2
Sunday	3.5	3.7	3.8	3.2
Shift:				
day	2.1	2.5	2.7	2.2
evening	3.3	3.5	3.3	2.6
night	3.5	3.3	3.4	3.0

Conditions of Nurses' Employment Contributing to Vacancy and Turnover

This section is intended to depict some of the conditions that could be viewed as contributing to potential dissatisfaction among nurses and hence could be construed as contributing to potential vacancy and turnover. The variables available for this purpose include salary levels, the extent to which salaries have increased during the previous year, and valuation of the fringe benefit package available to nurses employed in the particular institution. It should be noted here that, due to the nature of this survey (one of institutions rather than individual nurses), it is not possible to ascertain directly either the relative importance of these factors to vacancy/turnover or the role that other variables (inflexibility of schedules, lack of autonomy, and the like) might play in the process.

The basic data are presented in Table 11.8, which shows, for each sector by level of nurse preparation, the median hourly salary for newly hired nurses (first panel); the percentage increase in that variable during the past year (second panel); the value of fringe benefits relative to average annual salaries (third panel); and the extent to which the responding facility felt that selected elements of its overall fringe benefit packages were competitive with those offered by other employers of nurses (fourth panel). The salary data shown for temporary staffing agencies are not comparable with those for the other sectors in that they represent the average hourly rate paid to all nursing employees, which vary rather considerably according to shift, assignment, and sector of temporary employment for the individual nurse.

In terms of both salary levels and the recent increases in salary offered to nurses, home health agencies in had an apparent advantage over the remaining three sectors. Average hourly pay for RNs employed in that sector was anywhere from $.80 to $1.28 greater than elsewhere, while the margin for LPNs ranged from $.50 to $2. Regardless of the level of nurse preparation, average salaries in home health agencies had risen at a faster pace than they did in other segments of the industry, with pay increases in nursing homes clearly lagging. Additionally, the nursing home sector, along with temporary staffing agencies, offered a less substantial fringe benefit package than did other employers, especially hospitals.

Compared with nursing homes and home health agencies, hospitals reported a higher degree of "competitiveness" with regard to nearly all elements of the fringe benefit package. More than three quarters of all hospitals indicated that their vacation plans, sick and holiday pay, retirement plans, and health and life insurance programs were competitive. While comparable levels of satisfaction were reported by nursing homes and home health agencies with regard to vacation plans, sick pay, and holiday pay, the degree of competitiveness was judged somewhat lower with regard to the remaining elements, especially among nursing homes. In this context, it should perhaps be noted that all of these benefits, with the exception of life insurance plans, were judged to be the most critical elements in a fringe benefit plan by each of these three employing sectors.

In addition to those benefits related to leave and insurance, a good fringe benefit package that will serve to reduce vacancy and turnover rates as well as strengthen efforts at recruitment of additional staff should incorporate provision for career advancement through continuing education. In this respect, hospitals again emerge as offering, in their opinion, a more consistently competitive benefit package to their nurses than is provided to their colleagues employed in nursing homes and home health agencies, especially with regard to educational leave, tuition reimbursement, and scholarship assistance.

TABLE 11.8 Salary and Fringe Benefit Levels for Professional Nurses, by Type of Employing Institution, 1988

Measure	Hospitals	Nursing Homes	Home Health Agencies	Hospices	Temporary Staffing Agencies
Median beginning hourly salary:					
RNs	$10.47	$9.99	$11.27	10.01	$16-29*
LPNs	$7.14	$8.63	$9.13	7.75	$14-15*
NAs	$4.67	$5.04	NA	NA	$7-8*
Median percentage increase in beginning hourly salary:					
RNs	8	5	9	8	NA
LPNs	7	5	11	8	NA
NAs	6	3	9	8	NA
Percentage of salary represented by fringe benefit package:					
RNs	25	16	21	22	15
LPNs	26	16	18	20	17
NAs	26	17	23	25	15
Percentage of employers considering fringe benefit elements as being competitive with remainder of industry:					
vacation	90	79	78		
sick pay	88	72	72		
holidays	88	75	79		
retirement	76	29	50		
health insurance	79	63	72		
life insurance	82	60	67		
disability insurance	41	25	41		
personal leave	71	59	64		
educational leave	53	33	28		
sabbatical	10	11	9		
tuition reimbursement	70	53	46		
scholarships	34	20	13		
paid conference time	31	54	57		
paid CEUs	67	57	64		

*Range shown varies according to shift, nurse specialty, and sector of employment.

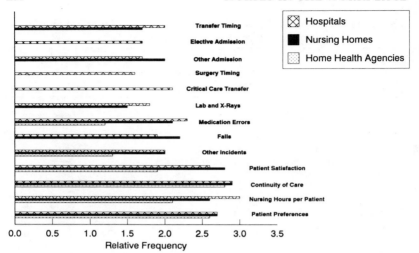

Figure 11.3. Frequency of Need to Deviate from Established Standards for Selected Procedures Due to the Nursing Shortage
NOTE: Data are mean values of a five-point scale, where 1 = not at all and 5 = very frequently.

Institutional Responses to Shortage

The responses to problems of shortage and turnover were measured in the survey by data reporting deviations from established standards; expenditures for overtime, temporary staff, and recruiting; and use of a wide variety of strategies available to reduce vacancy and turnover and, at the same time, to enhance the attractiveness of the institution to potential new employees.

We would include under the rubric "deviations from established standards" the need to close, at least temporarily, some of the facility's beds during the preceding year as a direct result of a shortage of nursing personnel. Some 15% of hospitals, but only 2% of nursing homes, indicated that they had been forced to take this comparatively drastic step. A wide array of other deviations from standards were reported, however. Each reporting hospital, nursing home, and home health agency was asked to indicate, on a scale of 1 ("not at all") to 5 ("very frequently") the extent to which specified deviations occurred. These are summarized in Figure 11.3. For hospitals, deviations in terms of the number of nursing hours per patient, continuity of nursing assignments, and responsiveness to patient preferences were reported to occur on a frequent basis. Nursing homes reported frequent deviations for each of these three items as well as for overall patient satisfaction. For home health agencies (where many of the items included are largely irrelevant or inapplicable), continuity of assignment and responsiveness to patient preferences were singled out as areas of special concern.

The use of temporary staff, enlisted either from in-house pools or from temporary staffing agencies, was quite common among both hospitals and nursing homes: 79% and 67%, respectively, reported at least an occasional use of temporary nurses during the survey year. This was also the case for slightly more than one fourth of the home health agencies. Slightly more than half of all hospitals that hired temporary nurses used an in-house pool, and 90% indicated that they made use of a temporary staffing agency. Many institutions clearly made use of both these sources of temporary help. Outside agencies were also quite commonly used by nursing homes, with more than two thirds of these facilities that hired temporary staff using this device. Only about one fifth made use of in-house pools. Among the relatively few home health agencies that engaged in temporary hiring, about three fourths used an in-house pool and about half used an outside agency.

The widespread use of temporary nursing staff entails a considerable expense to health care providers. The average hospital that provided data on these expenses indicated an outlay of $730,000 for persons recruited from in-house pools and $568,000 paid to temporary staffing agencies. (Owing to differential response rates, these figures are *not* additive.) Consistent with the staffing patterns characteristic of hospitals, most of these funds were expended to hire temporary RNs. In the case of nursing homes, mean expenditures were some $45,000 for those hired through the relatively uncommon in-house agency and some $91,000 for those hired through outside agencies. Consistent with the staffing patterns characteristic of nursing homes, most of these funds were expended to hire temporary nursing assistants.

In addition to the hiring of temporary nursing personnel, institutions responding to the survey also reported expending significant sums on overtime payments to existing staff as well as for recruitment of additional staff. The typical hospital reported that it had spent nearly $300,000 on overtime, primarily to its RN staff, and

TABLE 11.9 Typical Expenses Incurred as a Direct Consequence of the Shortage

	Hospitals (dollars)	Nursing Homes (dollars)	Home Health Agencies (dollars)
Temporary staff	704,400	32,900	31,500
Overtime	297,000	55,400	21,400
Recruitment	89,700	11,200	16,800
Total	1,091,100	99,500	69,700
Per bed or per average daily census	4,900	829	820

almost $90,000 on recruitment. The typical nursing home reported expenses of some $55,000 and $11,000, respectively, with most of the overtime going to LPNs and NAs. For the typical home health agency, overtime expenses amounted to about $21,000, while recruitment cost another $17,000. In sum, if we assume that expenditures reported by responding institutions are typical of the experience of all institutions and if we adjust for the shares of institutions that indicated that they did *not* use one or the other of the sources of temporary staff, we would find the typical expenses incurred as a direct consequence of the nursing shortage that are shown in Table 11.9.

Many of the institutions shared with us some of the strategies they had chosen to employ to enhance their competitiveness in the labor market for nurses. These are summarized in Table 11.10. As a general statement, it can be argued that hospitals take a more aggressive posture toward both retention and recruitment than do either nursing homes or home health agencies. The proportion of hospitals employing the recruitment/retention strategies shown in the upper panel consistently exceeds that reported by the other sectors, often by rather wide margins. Thus, while practically all institutions included in the survey indicate that they have increased salary levels, a substantially greater share of hospitals indicate that they have improved the structure of their fringe benefit package, that they have adopted strategies allowing for more flexible work schedules, and that they have in place more mechanisms that promote increased educational opportunities for their nursing employees. Only with respect to alternative practice models do hospitals lag behind another segment of the industry (home health agencies) and, to a large extent, this may simply reflect the underlying differences in mission and organizational structure between these types of entities.

Hospitals also report a much wider range of activities designed explicitly to recruit additional nursing participation (lower panel of Table 11.10). While nearly all reporting institutions indicated that they employed newspaper advertising, a much greater proportion of hospitals also employed strategies such as career counseling for secondary and college students, out-of-state recruitment efforts, career days, participation at conventions, job fairs, and open houses. A much greater proportion of hospitals are affiliated with schools of nursing, which would tend to provide them with greater entrée to students graduating from these programs.

Discussion

Starr (1982) refers to the transformation of the U.S. health care system as the rise of a "medical-industrial complex" dominated by huge health care conglomerates and corporate chains. In the United States, for-profit chain hospitals are concentrated in the South and West, particularly in Florida, Texas, and California. Such institutions are generally medium sized, consisting of 100 to 200 beds (Starr, 1982).

In 1988, the national average distribution of hospitals was 14% for profit, 61% not for profit, and 25% publicly owned (American Hospital Association, 1988). Florida represents one area of the country where the for-profit health care industries have flourished. Approximately 48% of the 300 hospitals in the state are for profit (Florida Health Care Cost Containment Board, 1989; Serow & Cowart, 1990), an increase from 45% in 1987 (Florida Health Care Cost Containment Board, 1988) and 43% in 1986 (Florida Hospital Cost Containment Board, 1987). This is in contrast to 40% not-for-profit or voluntary acute hospitals and 15% public or state/locally owned acute hospitals (Serow & Cowart, 1990). Because of the relatively small size of proprietary institutions, 37% of acute hospital beds in the state are represented by the for-profit institutions, while the not-for-profit hospitals make up 47% of all beds in the state, and publicly owned hospitals, 16% (Florida Health Care Cost Containment Board, 1988). Three major national hospital chains own most

TABLE 11.10 Retention and Recruitment Strategies Employed by Florida Hospitals, Nursing Homes, and Home Health Agencies

Strategy	Hospitals	(percentage using) Nursing Homes	Home Health Agencies
Recruitment and retention:			
Salaries and benefits—			
increased salaries	98	97	91
increased salary range	96	85	84
child-care program	47	16	33
improved benefits	76	62	66
living with work	16	3	13
Career—			
nurse image enhanced	80	54	70
mentoring	55	22	39
job satisfaction surveys	71	51	61
career counseling	47	26	32
Education—			
internships	56	18	29
preceptorships	75	19	34
tuition reimbursement	92	67	57
in-service education	98	88	84
paid conference time	83	69	74
research involvement	27	7	16
computer training	44	11	22
Workplace flexibility—			
in-house registry	66	26	NA
weekend program	66	38	NA
part-time flexibility	93	79	85
10- to 12-hour shifts	88	44	NA
4- to 6-hour shifts	51	33	NA
clinical career ladders	47	36	38
Alternative practice models—			
case management	24	12	72
shared governance	25	13	28
work redesign	35	16	37
Recruitment:			
Recruitment center	25	17	10
Career counseling—			
junior high	49	28	19
senior high	62	39	25
junior college	62	43	36
college	62	37	41
Local education outreach	44	45	38
Job placement	37	67	44

TABLE 11.10 Continued

Strategy	Hospitals	(percentage using) Nursing Homes	Home Health Agencies
Recruitment—			
out of state	71	21	25
foreign	43	23	16
Career days	82	46	53
Advertising—			
direct mail	54	27	42
newspaper	98	92	93
radio/TV	28	20	23
Convention booths	66	32	53
Job fairs	77	37	44
Open houses for students	61	30	28
Counselor programs	36	17	16
Nursing school affiliation	82	54	41

of the 140 for-profit acute care hospitals in the state (Florida Health Care Cost Containment Board, 1989).

In 1988, 2% of Florida nursing homes were publicly owned, 12% not for profit, and 86% investor owned, and many of the latter are affiliated with national chains. The proportion of beds represented by each type of ownership closely followed the number of homes, largely because both the mean and the median number of beds for nursing homes is 120 beds (Florida Health Care Cost Containment Board, 1989; Serow & Cowart, 1990).

In examining the nurse labor market among for-profit, not-for-profit, and public institutions, we would expect that, by virtue of their association with national chains, for-profit facilities would have more employee career ladders, benefit packages, and opportunities for advancement, resulting in lower turnover levels. Although the relatively smaller size of for-profit institutions may contribute to fewer opportunities for specialty work and the higher salaries associated with specialty assignments, for-profit institutions are expected to show leadership in salary structures when compared with not-for-profit and public institutions.

We found substantial variation in these rates according to hospital ownership for both LPNs and NAs; in each case, vacancies were more acute in for-profit institutions (where nearly one fourth of budgeted positions were reported vacant) than in either public or not-for-profit settings. These differences were statistically significant. Although variation among RNs was minimal, analysis of variance showed that, in all specialty areas except operating room, vacancy rates were significantly higher in the for-profit sector. Similarly, turnover rates were noticeably higher in for-profit institutions, and the observed differences are statistically significant in every instance.

Similarly, there was substantial variation in vacancy rates for LPNs according to ownership, with vacancies being more acute in for-profit institutions than in public and not-for-profit settings. These differences were statistically significant. Turnover rates are much higher among NAs than among either RNs or LPNs. In each case, turnover rates are noticeably higher in for-profit homes, and the observed differences were statistically significant in every instance. These findings are consistent with the vacancy and turnover rates reported by Harrington (1991), in which proprietary institutions had higher turnover rates for nursing staff.

In terms of the average level of starting salaries in hospitals, it was only for LPNs that significant differences existed among ownership types; in this case, the starting salaries were significantly higher in publicly owned institutions than elsewhere. The percentage increase in average starting salary (for 1988 over 1987) offered to RNs and LPNs by for-profit hospitals, however, was significantly higher than that offered by public and not-for-profit hospitals.

In terms of the relative value of benefits provided for members of the nursing labor force, significantly higher levels were provided for both RNs and NAs who were employed in either the public or the not-for-profit sector. In terms of the *availability* of specific benefits at "competitive" levels (in the estimation of the hospital itself), significant differences occurred among ownership types for retirement programs and on-site day care, with for-profit hospitals significantly less likely to provide the benefit in question than were those publicly owned or operated on a not-for-profit basis. Similarly, for-profit hospitals were significantly less likely to be affiliated with a school of nursing and offered RNs significantly fewer steps on the career advancement ladder than did institutions with other forms of ownership. Not-for-profit hospitals employed significantly more RNs (per patient) than did other segments of the industry, although this finding may reflect differences in the intensity of care typically provided by the larger public institutions.

In terms of the average level of starting salaries in nursing homes, it was only for A.A. degree RNs and LPNs that significant differences did not exist among ownership types; for diploma and B.S.-level RNs, the starting salaries were significantly higher in publicly owned and not-for-profit institutions than among for-profits. Among NAs, starting salaries were higher only in publicly owned nursing homes. Furthermore, the percentage increase in average starting salary (for 1988 over 1987) offered to RNs and LPNs by for-profit nursing homes was significantly lower than that offered by public and not-for-profit nursing homes.

Finally, there are some differences in the behavior of hospitals in coping with nurse shortages as a function of their ownership status. For-profit hospitals are significantly more likely to use an outside agency to recruit temporary or part-time nursing personnel, although the average level of expenditures per hospital for outside agency supplied does not vary by ownership, presumably reflecting the smaller average number of beds for these facilities. The average dollar value of nursing overtime expense is significantly higher among not-for-profit institutions than in either for-profit or publicly owned hospitals.

Significantly higher levels of benefit value were provided for all segments of the nursing labor force who were employed in either the public or the not-for-profit sector. In terms of the *availability* of specific benefits at "competitive" levels (in the estimation of the nursing home itself), significant differences occurred among ownership types for retirement programs and paid educational leave. In each instance, for-profit nursing homes were significantly less likely to provide the benefit in question than were those publicly owned or operated on a not-for-profit basis. Publicly owned nursing homes were significantly more likely to be affiliated with a school of nursing and offered all nursing personnel significantly more steps on the career advancement ladder, although the difference was not significant for RNs. Finally, both public and not-for-profit nursing homes employed significantly more LPNs (per patient) than did the for-profit segment of the industry.

A contrasting pattern emerges in the nursing home. The average dollar value of nursing overtime expense is significantly higher among publicly owned and not-for-profit facilities than in for-profit homes, both in the aggregate and for LPNs and NAs.

Findings from this study indicate that vacancy and turnover rates of nurses in Florida hospitals and nursing homes vary by type of ownership, with proprietary employers experiencing higher rates than public or not-for-profit owners.

Our data demonstrate increased work load through use of overtime in both industries as well as increased RN to patient ratios in hospitals, particularly the not-for-profit institutions. For-profit hospitals more often used outside agency staff rather than overtime to augment their own staff to cover patient care needs in times of shortage. For hospitals, the shift to increased RN staff in not-for-profit institutions may indicate increasing intensity of the hospitalized patient population. For nursing homes, the increased ratio of LPN to resident population in the not-for-profit and public facilities may indicate downward substitution of LPNs for RNs during a period of RN shortage. This interpretation is supported by the significantly greater LPN overtime expense in these institutions. Thus a philosophical shift in levels of personnel for staffing may have permeated the not-for-profit nursing home industry during this period. One limitation to these interpretations is the lack of control of staffing ratios and overtime expense by size of hospital or nursing home.

Public and not-for-profit nursing homes reported significantly higher starting salaries, salary increases, and fringe benefits for all levels of nursing personnel. While fewer significant differences for these categories were seen in hospitals of different ownership, the trend of higher salaries was evident in public hospitals, higher raises in not-for-profit hospitals, and higher benefits for RNs and nursing assistants in both public and not-for-profit hospitals. The fringe benefit offerings of retirement plans and day-care support were consistently lower in the for-profit sectors of both industries. Because state-employed workers, including nurses, consistently enjoy a retirement plan contributed to wholly by the employer, this benefit alone may contribute to lower dissatisfaction with the workplace.

Our data demonstrate a trend of higher turnover rates in the corporate sector of both hospitals and nursing homes. The turnover rates for all levels of nursing personnel in for-profit hospitals significantly exceeds the mean turnover for all hospitals. In nursing homes, the turnover rates for LPNs and nursing assistants are significantly below the mean in both public and not-for-profit nursing homes as well as for registered nurses in public nursing homes (although to a lesser level of significance).

Consistent across both industries are patterns of increased work load evidenced by increased RN to patient ratios and increased expenditures for overtime pay. The corporate sector exhibited greater use of external temporary staff, which contributes to the transient nature of the nursing staff. Variables associated with job dissatisfaction (lower salaries, raises, fringe benefits, and retirement benefits) prevail in the corporate segments of both the nursing home and the hospital industries. In both industries, fewer opportunities for education benefits, affiliation with nursing programs, and career advancement opportunities via the ladder approach are found in the corporate sector.

Dramatic differences in turnover rates between corporate sector hospitals and nursing homes, and others, not only indicate serious problems in satisfaction and career development of nursing staffs but also negatively affect continuity and quality of care. From a business perspective, the costs of turnover are high and contribute to increased expense of labor in the form of recruitment, orientation, and supervision.

Dynamics of the Nurse Labor Market

Labor in our society has changed in recent years due to a declining industrial base and a movement to increased services. Service industries such as the hospitality industry, the leisure industry, and the health care industry often are labor intensive. Health care employs a large proportion of service workers because the industry is the third largest in the United States today, accounting for almost 12% of the gross national product and employing 5.5 million personnel.

The nursing pool in the United States is at 2 million, approximately 80% of whom are employed in nursing. The proportion of employed nurses is higher than the overall labor force participation of women generally. Because 96.5% of nurses are women, the high proportion of working nurses has an impact on the status of working women as well as on their own nurse labor market. Currently, 25% of the nurse labor pool is educated in associate degree programs. Three or four decades ago, the highest proportion were diploma prepared in noneducation institutional settings, but because those programs have closed and many nurses who were educated in diploma programs are retired, the proportion of practicing nurses with diploma education has declined to 40% of the pool. About 28% of the nurse labor pool is made up of baccalaureate-prepared nurses. Master's-prepared nurses make up less than 6.5%, and there are more than 5,000 nurses in the United States with doctoral preparation (*Seventh Report to the President and Congress*, 1990). When viewed in the context of total supply, however, it is an exceedingly small portion.

Some employed nurses are organized through unions. This varies from state to state, however, with major organized nurse collective bargaining units in Massachusetts, Wisconsin, Washington, Illinois, and New York. In the South, some Florida and Alabama nurses are also organized, but right to work laws influence the composition of the bargaining unit. In all, relatively few nurses, perhaps less than 100,000 nationally, are organized. Davis (1986) makes an interesting argument that the activities of organized labor during the 1930s and 1940s led to today's labor situation. The trends in nursing labor seem to have followed that of organized labor generally. In 1974, the American Nurses Association funded the development of local units in several states. In the 1980s, the power of organized labor in the United States began to decline in that local union leaders became less involved with the workers and more involved in negotiating contracts with administration that often serve to enhance the corporation (Davis, 1986). Negotiation of nurse contracts has moved in the same direction in that contracts for nursing units now emphasize fringe benefits, with prerequisites inexpensive to management such as educational leave and the provision of clinical ladder programs. Substantive changes in salary levels are not evidenced in current union contracts.

Looking at the pool of workers generally, we see more and more low-wage workers with fewer people working for fee reimbursement or for an annual salary. In the nurse labor force, the same practice follows, shifting from the early model of fee payments to nurses who were employed as private duty nurses to current trends of low-paid nurses, often employed on an hourly wage basis rather than with full-time annualized salary. The lower salaries tend to follow the practice of blue-collar workers rather than high-wage professions such as engineers. This has created a dependency on capital in the wage-earning labor force (Davis, 1986).

With the decline in unions, and particularly as women have left production activities and moved into clerical or service positions, unionization has not followed workers into these new occupations. Therefore the mass of secretarial, clerical, and service workers, who tend to be mainly women and low-wage workers, are usually not unionized. The absence of the advocacy of organized labor means that women wage workers tend to be dispersed and diffused throughout the labor market and do not have a spokesperson to advocate on their behalf for improving working conditions and for higher wages. It also means that employers have enhanced this disorganization among service workers by hiring more and more part-time employees so that the cost of benefits can be saved; labor then becomes a variable expense item, and workers will not group together on their own behalf. The high proportion of part-time and temporary staff in the health service industries benefits the employer not only in cost efficiencies but by diffusing the nurse labor force. Maintaining a large proportion of part-time employees and keeping wages low provokes the "churning" of the nurse labor pool even within a geographic area. This constant shuffling of personnel from one facility to another tends to weaken the control of labor—that is, nurses—in terms of determining their working conditions and also their salary and reimbursement. An interesting example of management control over the employee is the recent move by the third largest hospital corporation in the United States to sell a portion of its facilities to their employees as pension plan equity. This put the employees in a vulnerable position, in that the future viability of the pension plan is dependent upon their ability to operate and staff the hospitals in the most profitable manner.

Organized medicine has also fed into this changing labor scene for nurses by helping to promote the expansion of numbers of lower-paid employees. The recent proposal for the RCT (registered care technician—a low wage worker with short-term training and no opportunity for career advancement) as a substitute for registered nurses is a prime example of this form of downward substitution and creation of an ever widening cadre of low-paid service workers.

As health care has become more and more profit oriented and corporatized during the last few decades, there has been a shift in labor practices aimed at strengthening the position of management rather than that of the employee. For example, there have been moves to substitute by importing personnel—a prime example of management increasing the size of the labor pool, thereby keeping wages low because the foreign-trained nurse will work for a lower salary than the U.S.-trained nurse. Recent changes in immigration laws have helped promote this practice. Actually, the American

Nurses Association position to support the immigration laws was probably taken without considering the long-range impact of an expanded foreign nurse pool in the United States on the continued depression of wages for nurses.

Nursing does have an opportunity to initiate changes in the labor market. The health care system is undergoing significant upheavals, with mergers, diversification, and the "downsizing" of some of the largest corporations, many of which are not experiencing the profit margins of a decade ago. Nursing can continue to move into the ever expanding low-wage service worker category—and many nurses will be hired on a part-time basis—or it can position the profession to become a part of the high-wage or contractual services group. Whether there is a move to the high-wage, contractual wage group is going to depend on whether nursing develops new forms of practice and, more important, develops new relationships with capital. An example is the Baptist Hospital (Miami) model in which nursing services are organizing themselves similarly to a law firm with senior and junior nurse partners who have clerks and assistants working with them in a team effort. For nurses to retain control, the role of the nurse will need to be altered in the workplace and nurses will need to hire and supervise their own assistants who will work with them on a regular basis. Because we know that the low-wage labor force will expand, nurses will need to position themselves to be in control of the low-wage labor pool by hiring and supervising their own assistants and contracting with industry for the opportunity to deliver services at a professional level.

TWELVE

An Action Plan for Nurse Executives

CHARLOTTE C. DISON

Throughout the 1990s, there will be competition for nursing personnel between acute care, home health care, nursing homes, and public health. The pressures to control costs of providing care will continue to funnel patients from acute care settings into alternate care systems at an increasing rate. Technological advances will support providing an increased amount of care in the patient's home.

The nursing shortage will continue past the year 2000. The shortage is not only one of numbers of nursing personnel but one of appropriate qualifications. The shortfall of nurses is estimated to be more than 300,000 in the year 2000 (U.S. Department of Health and Human Services, 1990). Clearly, an action plan is indicated to provide quality nursing care in turbulent times. The nurse executive will provide the leadership and impetus to develop and put in motion strategies for successfully meeting the challenges. Clearly, it is a time for nurse executives to seize the day. The profession can be moved forward to attain important ⎯ ⎯als—value, prestige, and social and economic recognition.

While this plan is written from my frame of reference, which is acute care settings, the strategies can be applied in any of the four settings. The strategies that will be explored are

1. restructuring nursing care delivery
2. reorganization of hospital care delivery/decentralization
3. information system-supported patient units
4. creating a "futures" unit—a new paradigm
5. nurse-physician collaboration
6. increased autonomy/professional practice
7. collaboration with nursing education

Restructuring Nursing Care Delivery

The restructuring of nursing care delivery has historically focused most predominantly on nursing systems. The nursing department, the largest homogeneous population and the most labor intensive, has been the primary focus for restructuring. Nursing shortages especially drive the need to redefine the professional nursing role.

The two systems most commonly in use today are primary nursing and team nursing. Primary nursing, a concept developed by Marie Manthey, became popular in the 1970s. The benefits of primary nursing are that (a) it affords a professional model of practice, (b) the registered nurse achieves a degree of autonomy, and (c) consumer (patient and physician) satisfaction is high. With the advent of the prospective payment system in the early 1980s, primary nursing became the delivery system of choice. An all-registered nurse staff proved cost-effective both in reducing costs of care and in reducing patient length of stay.

Team nursing used the professional nurse to coordinate, plan, and deliver care through a team of caregivers, which included licensed practical nurses and nursing assistants. The team leader's skills and preparation determined the success of this concept. The benefits to be derived from team nursing were that the system was less RN intensive and used less expensive personnel who were less difficult to recruit. Team nursing is still in use and, in some cases, is being reevaluated as an alternative way to deliver nursing care.

Primary nursing was the system most frequently in use in the hospital study *Magnet Hospitals: Attraction and Retention of Professional Nurses* (McClure et al., 1983). In the replication of this study, *Beyond Shortage: Nursing Personnel in Florida* (Serow & Cowart, 1990), primary nursing was still identified as the predominant care delivery system most favorably affecting nursing satisfaction. The nursing shortage along with the higher salary costs of an all-RN staff have prompted innovations in this system.

Partners in Practice™ is an adaptation of primary nursing that was developed by Marie Manthey, the originator of the primary nursing concept (Manthey, 1988). Partners in Practice™ is a system that enables the use of assistive nursing personnel with the values of primary nursing left intact within the system. This includes having one registered nurse (a primary nurse) who is responsible for the planning and a portion of the delivery of the patient's nursing care, which provides continuity of care between caregivers and uses the registered nurse as the key professional in the coordination and delivery of the patient's nursing care. Partners in Practice™ was an idea born from the nursing shortage to enable the retention of primary nursing values yet evolve a less RN intensive system. This system was introduced in pilot hospitals across the nation in 1989. The pilot hospitals were Good Samaritan Hospital in Los Angeles, Good Samaritan Hospital in Phoenix, Baptist Hospital of Miami, and Barnes Hospital of St. Louis, Missouri.

Key features of the Partners in Practice™ system include the following:

1. The partnership will consist of a senior partner who is a skilled, experienced registered nurse and a practice partner who may be a graduate nurse, a licensed practical nurse, or a nursing assistant.
2. Partners in Practice™ has some nurse-empowering features inasmuch as the senior partner interviews and recommends for hire the practice partner.
3. The partnership carries a caseload greater than that of a single caregiver.
4. The partnership signs a nonlegally binding contract that incorporates their willingness to work the same tours of duty and be mutually supportive of one another (Manthey, 1988-1989).

Within the Partners in Practice™ system, there is an opportunity for advancement for the professional nurse as well as for the practice partner. The decision to form a partnership is voluntary on the part of nursing staff, who actually apply to be considered for advancement to partnership positions. The salary program for the partnerships not only incorporates an increased salary for this responsibility but enables the senior partner to earn a significant number of points to apply toward the clinical advancement process.

The Partners in Practice™ system is in use in multispecialty acute care units (medical-surgical units), obstetrics, and critical care areas. Nurse satisfaction with the system is high. Some practice partners have been encouraged to go to school to become licensed practical nurses or registered nurses as a result of the positive experience in the partnership program.

The implementation of Partners in Practice™ is dependent upon having a pool of experienced nurses who are interested in this concept as well as a pool of ancillary staff from which to draw. Preparation for implementation of the partnership program is a key to its success. This preparation occurs at both the management level and the clinical level.

It has been said that delegation is a lost art with clinical nurses. One of the first aspects of preparation of senior partners is an educational program that addresses values, work roles, functions, prioritizing, assignment, delegation, and follow-up. In addition, the senior partner takes classes in interviewing and selecting a practice partner and then in coaching, evaluating, and maintaining a healthy, productive partnership relation.

Once the partnership has been formed, there are also classes for the partnership. This provides an opportunity to understand the framework of the partnership and the expectations for both the senior partner and the practice partner.

Unit preparation for introducing Partners in Practice™ includes forming a unit-based staff management team to address staffing, assignment, and relationship issues that occur between partnerships and nonpartnered staff within the unit. The staff management team is essential to provide input into the effectiveness of the system as well as to assist in evaluation of the outcomes. The staff management team provides support to enable the success of the concept.

MANAGEMENT PREPARATION

Because the nurse manager's role is significantly affected by creating a distribution of authority in the form of the senior partner within the unit, preparation is essential. A management program that allows the nurse manager to examine his or her management style in relationship to the delegation of authority in creating a climate conducive to the partnership is important. The partnership concept will not work effectively unless it is fully supported at the nurse manager level.

Partners in Practice™ can be effective in enabling the delivery of a high quality of nursing care under a primary nursing framework while reducing the number of RNs required to deliver nursing care. Partners in Practice™ is a system that also enables the attainment of the standards for quality of professional practice as well as quality of patient outcomes. Partners in Practice™ provides opportunities for advancement economically and professionally for both the senior partners and the practice partners. The partnership offers an opportunity to evaluate the incorporation of other types of caregivers into the partnership mode. This is particularly true in specialty units, such as a pulmonary unit, where a respiratory therapist may be a permanent part of the staff of the unit. The opportunity to offer the partnership practice role to other types of caregivers is afforded in this model.

Another model to be considered is the case management model developed at New England Medical Center in Boston (Zander, 1988). In this model, a primary nurse case manager is responsible for patient care and outcomes throughout the entire episode of the patient's illness. A case management plan and protocol for specific case types—critical pathways—is used. This is linked with case-specific physicians.

Another model in use is the Pro-ACT™ model developed at the Robert Wood Johnson University Hospital (Tonges, 1989). This model incorporates a clinical case manager who begins to work with patients before they come to the hospital. The case manager links the primary nurse and an associate nurse into a system to provide continuity of care.

The clinical case manager is required to be baccalaureate prepared; the primary nurse is a registered professional nurse; and the associate, a licensed practical nurse. The clinical case manager manages the hospital stay of the caseload of patients, integrating care with that of other disciplines to ensure that patient outcomes are accomplished within the required time frame. The primary nurse provides both planning and assessment of patients' care as well as direct and indirect care for a caseload of patients. The associate nurse assists the primary nurse in carrying out the nursing care functions. The LPN functions as the associate nurse in this model and functions in accordance with the Nurse Practice Act under the supervision of a registered nurse. This model incorporates the restructuring of other patient care services to support decentralized care delivery at the unit level.

PITFALLS TO AVOID IN THE CARE DELIVERY MODELS
THAT USE ASSISTIVE NURSING PERSONNEL

(1) Ensure that assistive personnel are accountable to nursing. The delegated tasks must be consistent with the statutes of the state's practice acts.

(2) Ensure that the RN role is not reduced to tasks. The RN role is that of delegation versus assignment with emphasis on planning, coordination, and follow-up. Fragmentation should not reduce effectiveness.

(3) Systems should free the nurse to do cognitive aspects of care as well as some hands-on care. The nurse should not be tied to nursing the technology and paperwork.

(4) Nursing roles and functions should be based on education, competence, and experience, and nurses should be compensated accordingly.

Reorganization of Hospital Care Delivery/Decentralization

Patient care services other than nursing have typically been compartmentalized by function and centralized either to provide direct services to patients in a central location or to act as a central distribution point. Nursing has been organized along these same lines with the identification of patient units as nursing units. The focus has changed to the patient as the elemental level of service with clinical and material supports refocused to the *patient care unit*.

This concept is most clearly demonstrated in the patient-focused model, which is currently being implemented at Lakeland Regional Medical Center in Lakeland, Florida. Traditional services including radiology and pharmacy as well as environmental supports are organized to report to a clinical manager/coordinator of the unit. Care is delivered by "care-pairs," a nurse paired with another caregiver who may be a pharmacist, radiology technician, or other health care worker.

In this model, there is decompartmentalization of the lines between jobs to improve efficiency and delivery of care. The jobs performed are determined by type, skill level, and potential of the worker within the regulatory constraints, such as practice acts or standards for hospital licensure (Watson, 1990).

Another approach is to "satellite" key services to the patient care unit. This is particularly effective for pharmacy, respiratory therapy, and selected radiology and laboratory services. The proximity of these professionals to the physician and nurse can strengthen the patient care team and at the same time provide an opportunity to improve the timeliness and quality of services delivered.

The multifunctional or multipurpose worker is a creative approach to breaking down the traditional job lines to produce cross-trained, multiskilled workers. Multiskilling is occurring especially in support jobs. Some examples are these:

- unit secretary cross-trained as monitor technician
- patient care technician cross-trained as monitor technician
- patient care technician cross-trained with phlebotomy skills

The position of the multipurpose worker provides an advancement opportunity for both economic and personal growth for individuals in support positions.

Information System-Support Patient Units

There is an explosion of health care technology with the ability to rapidly generate clinical data. The challenge is to integrate and synthesize information into the patient's plan of care in a timely way. Nursing is the last clinical service to be fully automated. Priority has been given to financial and diagnostic services with order entry systems and results reporting the next to be implemented. As a result, nursing has seen an increase in paperwork—tracking, reading, synthesizing, reporting. As much as 40% to 60% of a nurse's time is spent in information-related activities. The nurse needs to be supported with technology that manages patient care information (Halford, Burkes, & Pryor, 1989).

In late 1989, a survey was conducted to determine the status of computer support to nursing (Caron, 1989). The survey was distributed to nurse executives of 315 Florida hospitals, with a response rate of 78 surveys, or 25%. The computer supports in place were as follows:

computerized order entry/results reporting	53.0%
computer support for nursing administration	70.5%
bedside (point of care) computer terminals	5.1%

The nurse executives considering installation of point of care computer systems constituted 45.6% of the sample.

Point of care systems are available in the marketplace. The expense as well as the limited ability of the technology to interface with other systems has slowed the implementation of computers at the patient's bedside. Increased computer support for nursing is essential. Computer support for nursing will become a recruiting and marketing tool. Commissions/groups studying future nursing needs are incorporating computerized patient care systems into their recommendations.

The effective nurse executive will develop a strategy to enhance computer support to nurses within the strategic plan for nursing services. Analyzing the benefits of the support, including the financial payback, is one strategy. Another is to determine whether the current in-house system can be networked and decentralized to a "nurse server" or mini-station supporting a small group of patients. The demands of an information age in health care, coupled with the increased value of nurses' time, strongly supports the integration of computer support into nursing care at or near the bedside.

Creating a "Futures" Unit— A New Paradigm

The nurse executive and the management team may choose to translate their vision into a prototype unit, which can incorporate features that support changes in care delivery as well as new practice models. At Baptist Hospital of Miami, an opportunity was presented when the decision was made to renovate patient care units that had been built in the late 1950s. The units were large: 65-bed units with semiprivate and ward accommodations, a central nursing station, and very limited support space in a central core. The nursing staff formed a project team to design the new units that would arise from the old. There were some architectural constraints, as the outward walls of the physical structure were to remain. An underlying tenet for the design was that it must support or enhance nursing care delivery near the bedside of the patient. Key features of the nurse-designed units included the following (Figure 12.1):

"Cluster" architecture: small decentralized patient care centers, two to serve 35 patients. The patient care center houses a hostess/unit secretary and serves as a communication center for the 17-18 patients housed in the cluster.

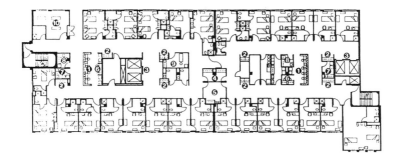

Figure 12.1. Five Main
SOURCE: Used by permission of TRO/The Ritchie Corporation, 3050 Bee Ridge Road, Suite A, Sarasota, Florida 34239; Patrick B. Davis, Jr., AIA, Project Director; and Fred C. Frederick, AIA, Project Architect.
NOTE: 1 = patient care centers (nursing stations), 2 = patient care stations (nurse servers), 3 = elevators, 4 = nurse manager/clinician office, 5 = conference room, 6 = physician's dictation, 7 = medication room, 8 = nourishment centers, 9 = respiratory therapy, and 10 = multipurpose room.

Decentralized computer/nurse/patient care stations: one for each four patient rooms strategically located adjacent to rooms served. The decentralized patient care station houses a CRT and computer terminal, nurse/call speaker, and telephone in addition to supplies and individual patients' medications. (All supplies including medications are delivered to the patient care station.) The computer has full capability for order entry, results reporting, and nurse care planning.

A progressive care unit: five beds especially designed for patients needing a higher level of care and technological support. The progressive care unit has telemetry capability for patients who require monitoring. The progressive care unit provides intermediate care support for those patients who do not need intensive care. This unit is a multispecialty acute care center, managing a variety of medical-surgical patients as well as developing a pulmonary subspecialty capability.

The model unit is supported by a satellite pharmacy as well as by respiratory therapy. The nursing system in place is Partners in Practice™. The staff are supported by a nursing management team and a full-time clinical specialist. The model unit has fostered nursing innovation and creativity. The unit will be used to study the impact of system redesign on nursing satisfaction, consumer (patient and physician) satisfaction, and effects on other health care disciplines.

Nurse-Physician Collaboration

As nurses gain more autonomy in nursing practice, the potential is great to exacerbate conflict between physicians and nurses. Further, the acuity of patients coupled with reimbursement pressures to reduce costs add to the tensions in relationships. The nurse executive must reckon with these issues to effect a positive relationship between the two groups.

One mechanism is to establish a collaborative practice network within the organization. This begins by gaining the support and endorsement of hospital administration, top nursing staff, and medical staff leadership. The Nurse-Physician Collaborative Practice Committee must be endorsed and supported by all three groups. One such model for a Nurse-Physician Collaborative Practice Committee has been established at Baptist Hospital of Miami. The mandate for the collaborative practice committee is a formal part of the medical staff bylaws and the nursing staff governance structure.

The purpose of the Baptist Hospital Nurse-Physician Collaborative Practice Committee is to enhance the working relationship between physicians and clinical nurses and the environment in which they practice. To this end, the traditional roles and relationships between physicians and nurses are critically examined by this committee to ensure the best use of skills and expertise of both professional groups and to promote a positive image. Although the interests of medicine and nursing diverge in some areas, there is considerable mutual interest in the central aspects of care.

The composition of the committee is a cross section of clinical nurses, physicians, and a nurse manager. The physicians on the committee are selected by the medical chairperson. The nurses are representative of the major nursing divisions and are selected by their peers with nurse manager approval. Membership on the committee continues for one year. The committee meets monthly and reports issues to the appropriate body, that is, the Medical Board or Nursing Council. There is a rotating chairmanship between nurses and physicians. Decisions are made by consensus.

To facilitate the selection of nursing staff who have both interest and skills to bring to the successful functioning of the committee, an application form was developed by the collaborative practice committee. The application form includes the following questions:

What do you have to offer to this committee?
What topics or issues would you like to see addressed?

The commitment to the appointment is then defined, and the applicant is asked to sign and to obtain nurse manager endorsement.

The interest level in the committee has been high. The committee meets on a monthly basis at a dinner meeting in the hospital board room. Activities of the committee have included addressing protocols that affect both medical and nursing practice, establishing protocols for independent nursing practice, and dealing with items such as communication issues.

Another way of involving physicians and nurses in collaborative activities is the appointment of nurses to medical staff committees. In some of these groups, quality assurance has been integrated to incorporate not only medical quality assurance but nursing quality assurance.

Unit-based joint practice committees also facilitate nurse-physician interaction. The critical care units have established a nurse-physician joint practice committee. This group deals with issues concerning nurse-physician relationships but has also addressed more far-reaching issues such as ethical matters and policies and procedures that affect the operation of the unit.

In other specialty areas, nurses are represented on the Oncology Executive Committee and the Family Birth Place Steering Committee, which is chaired by a rotation among nurse managers in that area. These endeavors have been quite productive in addressing the need for change or bringing about new developments in patient care services that affect both the physician and the nurse.

The Joint Commission on the Accreditation of Healthcare Organizations, in its 1991 standards for nursing services, strongly identified the need for nurse participation along with other leaders of the hospital including the medical staff in decision-making structures and processes. Included in this is the participation of the nurse executive and other nursing representatives along with physicians in the areas of planning as well as in quality monitoring and improvement

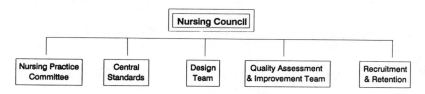

Figure 12.2. Shared Governance Organizational Model

activity (Joint Commission on Accreditation of Healthcare Organizations, 1990).

Steven M. Shortell, in his study *Effective Hospital Physician Relationships,* has suggested that the current trend will mandate that nursing plays an expanded role and will require a more collegial and equal relationship with physicians:

> Among other things this will require a greater amount of joint training of physicians and nurses in management skills including coordination, negotiation, problem-solving, and leadership approaches. In particular, medical staff and nursing staff leadership will need to work together to set the appropriate tone for the relationship and advance mutual interest. If the experiences of the present sites are any guide, it is unlikely that hospitals and physicians will be able to make much progress in the 1990s without active and ongoing nursing involvement, support, and leadership. (Shortell, 1990)

Increased Autonomy/Professional Practice

Nursing has been termed the last unliberated profession inasmuch as nurses work within a bureaucratic structure in which the nurse's formal authority does not extend beyond the actual delivery of nursing care. This compression is further aggravated by the unclear identity of the nurse within the system as relating to other power groups such as the physician. Nurses' inability to speak with one voice reduces effectiveness and often creates inability to reach consensus. Shared governance systems afford the nurse both the authority and the opportunity to influence aspects of practice that matter.

Shared governance is a system that moves beyond the concept of participatory management. Shared governance is based on the concept that there is a planned model for nursing input into decision making that affects not only the clinical environment but administrative and organizational issues. This philosophy begins with the nurse executive and flows through the administrative team and the entire staff. Shared governance structures may be set up around a council structure, which affords opportunity for input into and recommendations for decision making. One such model incorporates the following approaches: Unit-based management groups feed into a central process committee for clinical issues and to central standards committee for policy input and issues. All recommendations are then funneled to a Nursing Council for final review and decision making or for referral to an appropriate body (Figure 12.2).

The *Nursing Council* is the decision-making body for nursing practice within the hospital. The functions of the council are to

1. develop and approve policies to support uniform standards for nursing practice;
2. coordinate mobilization of resources to effect programs, policy, or problem resolution;
3. serve as the credentialing body for nurse professionals seeking privileges;
4. support total quality improvement by acting on issues affecting institutional nursing practice; and
5. review/approve recommendations forwarded to the council.

Representation includes the key nursing department head or manager from each area where nursing is practiced, chairpersons of the teams and committees, and nursing support professionals, such as in nursing education.

The *Central Nursing Standards Committee* coordinates development and maintenance of Generic Nursing Standards and integrates departmental and unit-specific standards to ensure a system for a uniform standard of nursing practice. Functions include

1. developing and maintaining Nursing Structure Standards and reviewing and/or revising them annually,
2. reviewing and approving Nursing Clinical Standards submitted by the Nursing Practice Committee, and
3. acting as a resource to other departments to synchronize nursing practice.

Membership consists of the chairperson, a nursing administrator appointed by the vice president; the cochairperson, a nursing quality assessment (QA) coordinator; vice president of the Patient Care Division; chairperson, Nursing Practice Committee; and six directors of nursing or their representatives.

The *Nursing Practice Committee* develops, maintains, and recommends for approval clinical practice standards and provides guidance to departments in the development of unit-/department-specific practice standards. Some key functions include

1. identifying generic and unit-specific standards to be developed;
2. developing clinical practice standards consisting of procedures, protocols, guidelines, preprinted nursing care plans, and discharge nursing instructions;
3. researching and recommending a procedure book to be adapted for basic procedures;
4. selecting and adapting procedures in the procedure book to be used in nursing departments;
5. reviewing clinical practice standards annually and revising as indicated;
6. making recommendations to nursing education/adjunct faculty regarding the education of the staff in new practice standards; and
7. providing guidance to department/unit standards committees in development of unit-/department-specific standards.

Recommendations from the committee are to be routed as follows:

- Generic forms and new standards are to be submitted to Central Standards Committee for approval.
- Unit-/department-specific standards are to be submitted to the appropriate nursing department director and then to the vice president for approval.

Membership includes clinical representatives from the patient care division including medical-surgical, obstetrics, critical care, special care, nursing education, patient education, patient treatment center, and dialysis; representatives from other departments such as emergency and rehabilitation; and others as needed. The chairperson is elected from the group and is approved by the department director and Nursing Central Standards Committee with a term of two years.

The Design Team plans the nursing care delivery model(s) with particular emphasis on Partners in Practice™. The team develops the framework for implementation, monitors the project, and develops revisions and innovations. Some examples of its work include developing criteria for selection and performance standards for the senior partner and practice partner and developing evaluation criteria for the partnerships.

Membership includes clinical, managerial, and educational staff. The team is chaired by the coproject director for Partners in Practice™.

The *Quality Assessment and Improvement Team* has monitoring and evaluation functions decentralized to the unit level, where there is one nurse appointed to be responsible for coordinating the monitoring and evaluation activities on that unit. Peer review is used to evaluate the quality of nursing care given.

Unit-based nursing representatives form the QA and I Team for the nursing division. Reports and recommendations are funneled to the Nursing Council.

The *Recruitment and Retention Committee* serves to promote recruitment and retention of nursing staff and fosters communication channels between nursing staff and the committee. An annual nursing satisfaction survey is conducted through the auspices of this committee, and the results provide a basis for the committee's activities. Some examples of work include establishing guidelines and incentives for floating, planning and supporting Nurse Week activities, and recognizing staff through the unit Nurse of the Year program.

Collaboration With Nursing Education

The most common relationship between nursing service and nursing education programs is that of affiliation of students into the practice setting for clinical instruction and experience. Nurse executives have great interest in the development of the student, for he or she is part of the future nursing staff. The shortage of nurses has had its impact on the supply of prepared faculty. The other constraint schools face is that of funding. Collaboration and cooperation between nurse executives and educators can be beneficial in meeting the mutual objectives of each.

Nursing service has increasingly attracted master's-prepared and some doctorally prepared staff. Joint appointments and shared employment between the educational institution and the hospital can provide expert clinical faculty. Another approach would be for the educational institution to contract with the hospital to provide qualified clinical instructors, subject to meeting the standards and qualifications for academic appointment.

Bringing academic programs to the work site is another way of strengthening service-education linkages by offering a convenient opportunity for staff to advance their credentials. One example is the LPN to RN transition program that may be offered in alliance with a community college. The course of study is part-time and spans two years.

Another program is the RN to B.S.N. completion program. More than two thirds of the registered nurses graduating today are from associate degree programs. The RN to B.S.N. completion offered at the work site affords an opportunity for nurses to enhance their knowledge and credentials. These programs are frequently coupled with tuition assistance offered by the employer.

The service agency may also offer clinical appointments to faculty to afford an opportunity for clinical practice, special projects, or research. One example is a faculty member developing and coordinating the summer externship for students in a local hospital. The faculty member can design the course so that it can be offered for college credit through the university nursing program.

Summary

The nurse executive is challenged today by multidimensional problems in maintaining a qualified and highly motivated nursing staff. Pressures to reduce costs of health care have led to greatly shortened lengths of stay and, as a result, increased acuity of patients who require more, not less, nursing care. The nursing shortage has left fewer nurses to meet the demands. What results is a fast-paced, highly stressful environment that can take its toll on the nurse in the form of lowered morale or attrition to a less stressful job.

The strategies described in this chapter can be used successfully to create a climate for professional nursing achievement. Nursing staff are integral to the success of the health care agency and its product: quality patient care. Quality nurses are difficult to recruit and difficult to retain; however, involving the nurse fully in the enterprise of patient care can have excellent results—for the nurse, the employer, and the patient.

THIRTEEN

Changes in Institutional Care Delivery: The New Role of the Nursing Professional in the Redesigned Workplace

PETER J. LEVIN

BARBARA J. CLARK

The basics of delivering care to sick people are often forgotten in the midst of issues confronting twentieth-century health care in America. During the 1980s, spiraling health costs encouraged widespread adoption of managed care in both public and private sectors. Managed health care products and programs are likely to remain popular in the 1990s; however, they do not appear to have been as successful in controlling costs as had been expected. The percentage of the health care work force employed both by health maintenance organizations (HMOs) and by providers contracting with preferred provider organizations (PPOs) continues to increase and is expected to be a substantial portion of the health care work force by the end of the 1990s (Findlay & Silberner, 1990). This is particularly important for physicians because the fee-for-service model for delivering care will decrease in importance in the years ahead. Controlling medical costs by reducing inappropriate care may be one of the best ways to solve this problem. Dr. Arnold Relman, editor of the *New England Journal of Medicine,* and other experts have stated that rationed care may be the unsettling alternative to this problem (Findlay & Silberner, 1990).

AUTHORS' NOTE: We thank John D. Thompson, Professor Emeritus of Nursing and Public Health at Yale University, for his suggestions on the content of this chapter.

235

Only now, with health care costs appearing uncontainable and with a shortage of nurses in selected specialties and localities, is the nature of the nurse's role in health care organizations being seriously challenged. Nurses have become even more essential for hospital operation than ever before. Yet they do not hold the power or authority necessary to command inclusion in the hospital decision-making process. Once again, there is a perceived shortage of nurses. We have been through nursing shortage crises regularly since the end of World War II. In the past, the answer was simply to expand nursing schools and to pump out more graduates. Today, the remedy does not appear to be that simple, especially when nursing no longer is viewed as a particularly desirable career for women. It will become necessary to create a health care environment in which the nurse has a series of roles and career opportunities open to her or him, which have clear career pathways with room for professional and self-growth, and adequate increasing remuneration.

The role of nurses in institutions has changed over time. Decades ago, hospitals were primarily staffed by registered nurses (RNs) assisted by student nurses and by orderlies. As time went on, new fields of various kinds were created as the need for special skills grew. The knowledge base and the technical competence necessary for the creation of new types of health professionals developed, and more staff took on functions that previously would have been carried out by nurses. Professions such as laboratory technology, physical therapy, and respiratory therapy evolved when nurses could no longer perform these functions as part of their routine duties.

At the same time, nursing education itself went through a series of changes. The three-year, hospital-based diploma school was being phased out to be replaced by the four-year university baccalaureate program. Before the bachelor's degree became the replacement for the diploma, community colleges developed two-year associate degree programs in nursing and quickly became the major producers of registered nurses in the country. The reasons for these changes in education have never been fully accepted in the hospital and medical worlds and tend to be overlooked by the general public. Nursing educators believed that the bachelor's-prepared nurse should become dominant, and therefore they wished to end the three-year hospital training schools. Now, the three-year training school based in the hospital has virtually disappeared and, in many instances, the four-year collegiate programs are hard pressed to fill their classes.

Several questions come to mind. One must ask: For what are these associate degree nurses being trained? Is a two-year curriculum at the community college level comparable to three years in the work setting or four years in a collegiate atmosphere with a much heavier emphasis on basic science? If there are real differences in curricula between these programs, what is missing and what should be changed or added? Should a nurse function only as a nurse, or are there additional pathways for which a nurse should be trained beyond his or her first degree, whether obtained from a two-year community college or a four-year bachelor's program? Why hasn't the concept of an internship period after licensure ever been promoted?

Nursing, as a profession, has continued to evolve since World War II with increasing opportunities for nurses to specialize in clinical or other areas. Nurse practitioners, certified nurse midwives, clinical nurse specialists, nurse researchers employed in clinical settings, and primary care nurses have evolved because of the need for nurses trained with specific skills. In addition, nurses have moved into new roles developed within the health care system, roles that have been assigned to them and for which they have been deemed competent. Included in these areas of new responsibilities and skills are quality assurance, infection control, risk management, IV teams, hemodialysis, information systems, discharge planning, and case management. It is important to emphasize that many of the additional tasks within these roles that have been assigned to nurses were not and still are not part of the curriculum of nursing education.

The overlap of duties among health professionals makes it difficult to handle nursing shortage issues without considering the supply of workers in other closely related fields. For example, the overlap between specialized nurses and physicians has affected the use of nursing resources in these expanded roles. The ways in which these resources are affected depend first on the supply of available physicians, nurse practitioners, and certified nurse midwives and, second, on the attitudes of physicians, employers, legislators, third party payers, and consumers toward use of these nurses. These groups can dramatically affect such things as criteria for licensure of nurses, availability of malpractice insurance, payment for services, and employment practices. A good example of this effect is the allowing of prescriptive authority by nurses in nursing homes in the absence of physicians. Thus the nursing shortage has become a more far-reaching and complex issue than one would have initially suspected.

One of the areas of greatest importance for the future management of health care in the United States is the ability to fully recognize and integrate nursing management into both institutional and out-of-hospital care. Recently, the nurse's role has been slowly evolving into one of managing patient care activities (Dittrich et al., 1979, cited in Revicki & May, 1989). Within this changing role, the managerial responsibilities may include supervising other nurses and ancillary personnel plus accomplishing a wide range of organizational, patient care, and personal objectives. Some nurses provide bedside care while others manage multimillion-dollar budgets. Rarely is the nurse thought of as a management person, yet, frequently, nursing service is often the largest labor component in a hospital's budget (Aiken, 1989). This being the case, what preparation and recognition should be given to the variety of nurse managers? Somehow this issue regarding nursing preparation has been less satisfactorily addressed than have the changes in education for physicians and hospital administrators. This is strange because nursing is central to the delivery of care in the hospital, nursing home, and a variety of other institutional and noninstitutional settings. No one has come up with a professional who can replace the nurse. The recognition of this is long overdue.

Society has behaved very strangely in its expectations of the nurse. On one hand, patients want a caring, concerned individual at the bedside and, on the other hand, organizations require someone who is a highly trained technical expert, with the ability to make judgments about an individual's condition based on firsthand observation. At the same time, these individuals also are supposed to be promotable into management positions, where there is constant conflict between their roles as healers and their roles as managers. While this dichotomy has always existed, cost issues and management issues around staffing and providing care have come to dominate much more of our health care system. The technology nurses are expected to master has gone far beyond taking the pulse, temperature, and blood pressure. For example, titrating drugs and complex cardiac and other equipment requires an understanding of the pharmacology and physiology of various bodily systems and functions, to facilitate making judgments about changes in condition and therapy. U.S. community hospitals have nurses on staff around the clock who are expected to monitor the condition of the patient, deal with the orders and the preferences of physicians, and be independent professionals making correct judgments for the patient, the institution, and themselves.

Although these tremendous demands, complexities, and responsibilities are recognized within the nursing profession, studies have shown the public's perception of nursing to be somewhat different. Research regarding society's image of nursing comes from two sources: studies of public opinion and analyses of mass media messages (National Center for Nursing Research, 1988). Evidence from public opinion polls, television, and other mass media has suggested that society perceives nursing as a low-status women's occupation that is not appropriate for men and that is lacking in money, autonomy, and power. It is probable that one unfortunate outcome of this deficient perception has been to produce low self-esteem among nurses, making them feel undervalued and that their work is unimportant. And so the nursing shortage is fueled from yet another source. It must not be forgotten that nursing is an occupation with many inherent conflicts, and often is beset by stress, frequent job turnover, and early burnout. Finally, and fortunately, the long arm of malpractice rarely settles on nurses as individuals, probably because there is very little for which to sue because it is impossible to become rich while working as a nurse in America's health care institutions today.

Seriousness of the Shortage

It is interesting to note that, even though the supply of registered nurses has grown rapidly during the last decade, a very real shortage of nurses currently persists, and health care providers have had to adjust the way services are delivered. The types of adjustments to the delivery of services made by hospitals because of vacant nursing positions have been documented (Roberts, Minnick, Ginsberg, & Curran, 1989). At least 85% of hospitals have made some internal management and/or patient service adjustments due to the nursing shortage. When these measures fail, admissions are delayed, units are understaffed, or units may be closed temporarily.

GROWING DEMAND FOR NURSES

The current nursing shortage is demand driven and appears to be due to an increase in the number of additional nursing positions offered by hospitals. Nurses are drawn to more competitive hospitals, which has resulted in substantial shortages in less competitive care facilities, especially during the unpopular shifts. Additionally, leaders of organized nursing have been working to enhance nurses roles and their image. Some leaders have urged all-RN staffs for hospitals.

In looking at the growing demand, a prominent factor emerges. More and more biomedical and other technology has been added to the hospital workplace, which has resulted in a very high intensity of care and the need for highly trained personnel at the bedside to use this complex technology. Furthermore, the total number of very sick hospitalized patients has increased.

Changes in health care finance policies, particularly the Medicare and Medicaid prospective payment system, have put increasing financial pressures on hospitals in recent years. One result is that the length of stay is shorter. Also, it has encouraged outpatient care for less serious procedures. One asks then: How does this affect the demand for nurses? The introduction of the prospective payment system has resulted in an increasing trend toward substituting RNs for LPNs when the difference between the market wage rates for the two types of nurses is narrow and RNs are more versatile (Aiken, 1989).

America is aging, and its people are living longer. The baby boom generation is getting older and, with fewer young persons, the U.S. population is becoming top heavy. This trend is evidenced by a dramatic 4.4% increase in Florida's over-age-65 population during the 20 years from 1970 to 1990; and it is projected that, by 1995, 19.8% of its population will be 65 years and older (Mittan, 1989). Not only will this group need more health care services, the intensity of these services is expected to increase as well.

It appears that what is fueling the increasing hospital demand for nurses is likely to continue for years to come. The fact remains that the population is continuing to age, and there is little likelihood that it will become healthier. Disease prevention and public health measures are still being given second-class status to treatment procedures in the health care and insurance industries. And so, for the foreseeable future at least, hospitals will remain under pressure to employ more and more nurses.

THE DECREASING SUPPLY

The increasing complexities and demands of the nursing profession, without major changes in compensation, benefits, recognition, or other rewards normally found for employees in other sectors of our economy, have helped to fuel the shortage problem. Why is nursing caught in such a situation? The fact is that nursing is still widely accepted as "women's work" despite its competence at handling high technology and responsibility for providing care in the most extreme circumstances. There are still widely accepted shibboleths around the role of the nurse that have prevented it from changing in the way that many other professions, and nonprofessions as well, have evolved over time. More recently, the nursing profession itself has pushed for its own brand of professionalization, which it sees as a way to increase the status of nurses.

One can argue that public policy and changes in reimbursement policy have affected the availability of nurses by influencing wages. Comparison of nurse salaries before and after Diagnostic Related Groups (DRGs) has been documented (Aiken, 1986; Aiken & Mullinix, 1987). Before the Medicare prospective payment system (PPS), increases in nursing salaries were comparable to salaries of other hospital employees, whereas, after the implementation of PPS, nursing wage increases lagged behind those of other hospital workers. It has been suggested that some of the savings under DRGs came from the lack of adjustment in nurses' wages. And because nursing service often constitutes a significant portion of hospitals' budgets, it is an obvious target when budget reductions are required. Therefore the effect of policy changes on nurses' incomes cannot be ruled out.

Physicians and nurses must be part of a team in which they each have a right to independent decision making within broadly agreed upon, jointly compiled, guidelines. This is the way of the future in health care and it can be implemented quickly in specialized care units and in ambulatory care settings. More recognition of the importance of nursing care through true team care and higher pay will help to lessen dissatisfaction—but only after significant role change.

CHANGES IN OPPORTUNITIES FOR WOMEN

General acceptance of the traditional role of the nurse in the hospital, nursing home, and public health agency has caused little change even though there has been a constant outcry about the importance of nurses and their shortage. Salaries have finally started to increase. Change was slow not only in the rate of remuneration but also in the rate of recognition and integration of nursing into the very basic planning and administration of institutions. The rise of the investor-owned hospital movement in the United States during the 1970s and the mimicking of their competitive behavior by voluntary hospitals has not resulted in a fundamental change in the way care is delivered or in the importance of the nurse.

Due to this inertia in bringing about change, women began to seek careers outside of the traditional areas of teaching, nursing, and secretarial services. In the early 1970s, medical and dental schools began increasing the number of women students. The explosion of computer technology and the expansion of law, finance, and accounting resulted in many high-paid professional positions opening up for the first time to women. In retrospect, the 1970s would have been a good time to have made profound changes in the role of the nurse given that nursing had begun to lose its attractiveness to women as a career choice and hospital finances were able to support experimentation and innovation.

With these difficulties to overcome, hospital administrators began to look for viable solutions to the nursing shortage. A recent nationwide survey of 450 hospital administrators reveals that almost half of the administrators are implementing internal programs such as using support personnel to relieve nurses of nonnursing duties, providing competitive pay scales and shift differentials, and extending the hours of part-time nurses (Jensen, 1988). In addition, in an attempt to keep nurses on staff, administrators are offering tuition assistance and are encouraging nurses to pursue advanced degrees.

In rating the severity of the nursing shortage in their areas, hospital administrators reported a moderately severe situation, which is shown in Figure 13.1. At the same time, 1,000 consumers were surveyed to obtain their perceptions of the nursing shortage. Two thirds of the consumers surveyed said there is a shortage of nurses (see Figure 13.2). There was no difference between the perceptions of recently hospitalized consumers and those who had not been hospitalized.

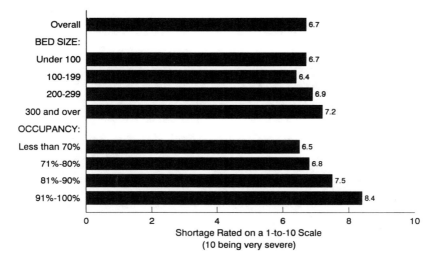

Figure 13.1. Hospital CEOs' Perspective on the Severity of the Nursing Shortage in Their Area
SOURCE: National Research Corp., as reproduced in *Modern Healthcare* (December 2, 1988). Reprinted with permission from *Modern Healthcare*; copyright Crain Communication, Inc., 740 N. Rush Street, Chicago, IL 60611.

Temporary Staffing Agencies

One available option that is being used to help alleviate the nursing shortage is that of the temporary staffing agency (TSA). Emerging as a controversial player in the market for nurses' services in the 1970s, TSAs compete with hospital float pools to provide nursing services. But are these agencies a solution to the problem of the nursing shortage or the problem itself? TSAs may become a long-term problem due to the "domino" effect: Higher use of these agencies results in the opening of more agencies, which results in a larger number of employers competing for the same pool of available nurses. On a positive note, TSAs can provide staff for critical needs. Serow and Cowart (1990) report that temporary personnel, from either TSAs or from in-house pools, were used by approximately two thirds of all of Florida's nursing homes and by more

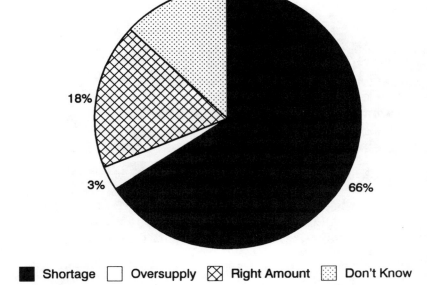

Shortage ☐ **Oversupply** ⊠ **Right Amount** ▦ **Don't Know**

Figure 13.2. Consumer Perception of Area Nursing Supply
SOURCE: National Research Corp., as reproduced in *Modern Healthcare* (December 2, 1988). Reprinted with permission from *Modern Healthcare*; copyright Crain Communication, Inc., 740 N. Rush Street, Chicago, IL 60611.

than 75% of its hospitals. This same source reveals that additional costs are incurred by nursing homes and hospitals when TSAs are used. As cost containment continues to dominate the health care scene, hospitals may be forced to decrease their use of temporary agencies in lieu of other more cost-effective measures.

The Hospital Environment

Nurses are essential for patient care because almost all basic care must be given by doctors and nurses. Without physicians and nurses, one cannot have a hospital. Physicians and nurses also help train other health care personnel to accomplish the tasks and objectives that only they can outline. In our more complex work-differentiated hospitals, many other health professionals augment this basic care. Despite the importance of the nurse in the patient-care setting, nurses' notes in the treatment of patients are rarely even looked at by physicians. The lack of importance of nursing notes to physicians and others demonstrates that the role that nurses occupy in the actual delivery of care is not as major decision makers in care delivery. While they observe the patient more than any other professional, theirs and others' observations do not drive the system.

The activities of nurses are not a by-product of the treatment process but are, or should be, the central focus of the routine management of the patient during the course of hospitalization. In a more efficient and streamlined system, the data revealed by nurses' notes, including the use of supplies and services, would be the central driving mechanism for the operation of the institution. The role of the nurse manager in orchestrating this process should have become much more paramount than it has in our system. It has not been usual and necessary for the nurse in hospital management to be considered a member of the decision-making management team. Despite the fact that nursing is critically important and that a large amount of money is directed through the nursing service, the importance given nurse managers in the triumvirate of medicine, nursing, and administration in the management and governance of the hospital is much less than that afforded the other two parties.

The necessity for competent nurse managers to manage the nursing budget has evolved slowly. The process of setting standards for the amount of care needed by patients, which depends on formulas and is put into operation through staffing patterns, remains little understood by hospital administration or the medical staff. These are viewed as nursing activities, and therefore it is not considered absolutely essential that they be understood and managed by those in charge of the overall operation of the hospital. Medicine and administration would not be expected to adjust their activities or control resources to support nursing ahead of central administrative or medical priorities. Intellectually, management has missed the importance of nursing for the hospital to be able to carry out its mission successfully.

Complexity surrounds the issue of what to do with the more highly educated nurse specialists. Accreditation requirements and advanced education for nurses have produced a staff top heavy with master's degrees, nurse specialists, and doctoral degrees.

Although advanced degrees denote expertise around clinical specialties such as pediatrics, geriatrics, psychiatry, maternity, and so on, what do they mean in terms of nurses' overall judgment for services management, and what role has been accorded them by the physician specialists in each of these areas? How has the hospital dealt with their additional expertise? Having advanced training by degree or certification is meaningful to nurses in the clinical setting, but what does it mean for hospital management and resource allocation or to the physicians who write the patient care orders? Why are some hospitals staffed with clinical specialists assigned to various services, and why is there no perceived need for them in other hospitals? Where does expertise in clinical care come in, and where is expertise in management needed? The nursing organizational structure in the hospital has done little to answer these questions.

The need to offer university education or advanced degrees is a U.S. phenomenon that follows the route of the development of professions and evolution of educational leadership. It is interesting that it does not appear to have answered the questions as to how helpful this truly has been to the elevation of the nursing profession in this country during the last several decades. Recently, nursing educators have played a limited leadership role in guiding change in the clinical setting. Nursing organizations have been strident for increased professionalism and for pay increases, which rarely have been satisfactorily resolved through collective bargaining.

The Nursing Home Environment

Nursing homes have served as the means of housing elderly people since society shifted from a rural to a predominantly urban environment and it became increasingly difficult for children to keep their parents on the farm or at home with them. This societal change allowed for the development of institutions that could accommodate the changes that occur physiologically, economically, or socially at the end of life. Initially, the bulk of this care was custodial, with the goal of maintaining people as healthy as possible for as long as possible. As this simplistic focus paralleled the general rise in longevity of the population, it became apparent that there was a need for a facility to provide posthospital care to patients who could be rehabilitated sufficiently to return to their own homes. This concept has grown, and nursing homes and other rehabilitation facilities are now serving this purpose. For the most part, the residents of nursing homes are there for the duration of their lives, and nurses play a key role in their health and in the management of the facility.

Traditionally, nursing homes were independently owned and comparatively small, 50 beds or less. As time has passed, large corporations have entered the nursing home business and the size of these institutions has grown. Most of the "hands-on" care is supervised by registered nurses who oversee the quality of care that is given to these patients, most of whom are long-term residents. Very few nurses, however, have significant training in long-term care and, more important, very few of them possess the managerial and motivational skills needed to be the captain of a team of persons with less education and motivation. The role of the nurse relative to caregiving and to management in long-term facilities must be rethought not only from the viewpoint of that of a manager of a large number of lesser skilled people but also on a work efficiency and task assignment basis. From the second perspective, it would be helpful, for example, if nurse practitioners were allowed to write prescriptions when overseeing nursing home patients. Long-term care is projected to grow and will take on increasingly complex patients, necessitating an expansion of the nurse's role within these facilities.

The Redesigned Workplace

It is time for hospitals to completely reorganize with the patient and the nurse in the center and all others surrounding them in a circular fashion. The physician is no longer the professional who knows the most about all patients. Patients are now categorized according to their disease, disabilities, and procedures needed for their treatment. The complex of people and equipment necessary for the performance of bedside care is being organized and approached from a more realistic managerial and statistical basis than ever before. One of the primary tools being used is the computer. The result is that a patient with a specific diagnosis or chief complaint and an array of physiological characteristics will have his or her treatment plan completed by a computer using information that normally will fit 90% of the people with that particular presentation. Staffing patterns and inventory control similarly can be derived. For the hospital to remain a human institution, the nurse, as the caregiver and supervisor of all care, must be in a much more pivotal patient managerial role than at the current time.

The notion that nursing is just another department of the hospital and acceptance of the concept that the physician is the initiator of all activity in the hospital are rapidly becoming obsolete. This does not mean to denigrate the physician's role as either a client of the hospital or the ultimate decision maker for patient care. Patient care decisions based on nurse's observations, however, must be given more validity. Because physicians no longer "live" at the hospital, it is the well-trained and experienced nurse who notes a patient's changing condition and, in the future, will recommend the technology to be used and changes in therapy. It will take some time for acceptance of this concept. Institutional organizations should be restructured so that the realities of patient care can be dealt with taking into account nurses' training and experience. This does not mean to supplant the physician in making diagnostic and treatment judgments but to consider the reality of the modern hospital and to recognize who really sees the patient the most. This will take a major change in physicians' attitudes in the inpatient setting, but this change will occur as more diagnosis and treatment takes place outside of the hospital and it becomes the focus of procedure-oriented specialty medical care. Recuperation and convalescence, even now, are taking place elsewhere, with little physician participation.

The New Role of the Nursing Professional

In this newly designed environment, nursing will be divided between those who give bedside care, those who have specialized clinical knowledge, and those who manage the system. Having undergone nurse's training, these employees must also possess the appropriate advanced training commensurate with their level of responsibility for decision making either as caregivers or as line managers. The high-tech nurse should be rewarded for his or her skill and competence and not be forced into a management position to receive a higher level of pay. Clinical experience and judgment should be recognized and rewarded by a reorganization of pay scales according to level of responsibility. This may result in the creation of various levels of nursing specialization, perhaps acknowledged by outside specialty board-type criteria that are tied to pay scales. These should be more than institution specific and should be transferable across nursing settings. Clinical ladders are one strategy being used by hospitals to give nurses more control and authority at the bedside. As such, ladders recognize the competence, education, and tenure of bedside nurses by granting them financial rewards and other benefits.

It is interesting to note the success of nurse practitioners and clinicians who already operate in a variety of outpatient care settings where physicians formally transfer authority commensurate with the nurses' levels of competence. This has been done successfully in the fields of psychiatry, midwifery, geriatrics, and pediatrics, all of which allow nurse practitioners to make judgments about the condition of patients and make changes in therapy. This currently limited perspective should be applied to a wider variety of settings, and the use of nurse clinicians in the hospital would be better served by more standardization and the development of career ladders across the field. This must occur not only to improve patient care and to acknowledge what is really taking place but also to allow for the emergence of nursing as a true profession with a career ladder and pay that is commensurate with the proper level of responsibility and accountability. Both hospitals and physicians would have to play a major role in this initiative.

In addition, nursing activities in all health care settings need to be managed by people who are skilled in management, budgeting, and techniques to improve efficiency and effectiveness. Few nurse managers have been taught the basics of counseling employees or group motivation techniques. More business applications need to be included in nursing education. The development of joint degree programs such as the RN-M.P.H. (Master of Public Health) and the RN-M.H.A. (Master in Health Administration) should be encouraged. At the same time, the goal is not to turn nurses into business people. Nursing, however, cannot continue along the current path with tremendous increases in responsibility and technical competence but only moderate value assigned to it in our society. Nursing is one of the oldest and certainly most noble of the professions, and it ought to be allowed the freedom and autonomy of other professions. People must be rewarded for being willing to care for others and be highly valued in our society for doing this. Pay scales and benefits of experienced nurses need to be overhauled and increased. Men should be encouraged to become nurses, and the rewards of such careers should be widely advertised.

It is not unrealistic to expect a couple, both of whom are nurse specialists, to have incomes and a standard of living similar to what might be expected by a couple in which both are attorneys. If we value good care at least as much as we value formal agreements between people, then we must reorder our priorities to achieve these results.

It is not expected that the hospital administrators of America will cheerfully and enthusiastically line up behind the proposed changes, which will be costly and disruptive. The proposed reorganization of the hospital will change the relationships between governing authority, administration, medicine, nursing, and patients. We are recommending a fundamental attitudinal change about the nurse-patient relationship and care given while in the hospital or nursing home. There must be more independent clinical judgment on the part of the nurse as well as more administrative competence and importance for nurses within each institution. Nursing no longer can be viewed as a series of tasks for which you hire someone with a particular license but should be seen as the foci of expertise within an individual. Nursing must contribute to the improvement of the health of patients and participate in the overall management priority setting of the institution.

Hospital administrators will have to change their outward-looking focus, which, while commendable, also insulates them from the realities of what is going on inside their own facilities in the provision of patient care. They must begin to look into their own institutions to better understand resource allocations and the reasons for them and then weld together a team of doctors, nurses, other professionals, and support personnel that really is focused on caring for the needs of patients.

This is not meant to thwart the current major focus on the bottom line, productivity, efficiency, and competition. We envision that, by using patient care as a focus, and by implementing management excellence, a win-win situation can be produced. Not only will the patient's health status be improved, and profits, productivity, and efficiency be increased, but enhancement of the nurse's role in the delivery of patient care will be achieved. This results in a positive image of the whole industry in the eyes of the public. Then and only then will real success be achieved. A new role for nursing in the redesigned health care workplace can come about with acknowledgment of the need for this change by hospitals, nursing homes, administrators, the medical and nursing professions, and the public. This is long overdue.

FOURTEEN

The Policy Agenda

MARIE E. COWART
WILLIAM J. SEROW

This study has contributed to a better understanding of the dynamics of nurse employment among various health care industries. The nursing personnel shortage that occurred at the time of this study was a significant one. It not only occurred at a time of widespread increasing demand for registered nurses and other nursing personnel, but it also occurred in concert with changes in women's participation in the labor force. Changes in female career choices triggered a decline in enrollments in nursing education programs as well. While these trends are well documented for nursing personnel, similar patterns were exhibited among other, allied health professions.

It is clear that rapid and extensive shifts in the health system and its regulatory structure during the last decade or so have resulted in reactive behavior on the part of health care providers in an attempt to address a discrepancy between the demand for patient care and the overall supply of health care workers. The reality of this imbalance is tempered with the awareness of changing preferences in career choices and in demographic shifts that will result in an overall reduction in the growth of the labor force. Thus a systemwide view of the overall problems of nursing personnel in the context of the entire health care industry is essential. In a word, *reform* of our traditional models of care, and uses of nursing and other personnel, is required to deal with the problems exhibited by the data from this study. There is a need to cease the reactive approach to the use of nursing personnel and to rethink the underlying purposes of our elaborate system of acute care hospitals, nursing homes, home care agencies, hospices, public health agencies, and other health services using these special care workers. A reemphasis on the individual, and the needs that emerge when the patient enters the health care system, is paramount. Such a reordering of priorities from the needs of the system, and its corporate owners, to the needs of the individuals in the society will provide a sounder focus for the use and demand for nursing and other health care personnel.

Given the prospects for increasing demand for health services and the future limitations of the supply of labor for health care personnel, systemwide reforms in the use of personnel are in order. This will require a focus on the elements of work involved in patient care and the discharge of the stabilized individual from the system. Such change cannot be accomplished successfully for nursing personnel alone but will need to include all levels and categories of health personnel, particularly those who work in concert with the nurse. The current fragmented system of acute and long-term care will become more effective and efficient through development of a coordinated care model that provides a continuum of services from prevention to acute and eventually long-term care. The health industries will need to redesign their respective organizational structures for this improved coordinated care, and the tasks to implement that care will need to be redefined. Such an overhaul may require job retraining and job redefinition, with implications for educational programs and professional licensure and reimbursement statutes. Protection of traditional roles and scope of practice for health professionals will need adjustment rather than protection of current disciplinary turf.

Because the need for reform of nursing and health personnel is widespread, such transformation will require thoughtful adjustment by all sectors now reinforcing the current demand for nursing personnel. Proposed widespread changes must start with the nursing profession for all levels of nursing personnel. The profession will need to assume leadership in defining and demonstrating innovative practice models for nursing personnel, which show the fit within the system and the benefit to the health care industry. Such models will need to demonstrate efficiencies in staff as well as quality enhancements and revenue contributions. The fit of these models with other disciplines will need to be clarified. Such models will need to strengthen nursing's role in clinical decision making to provide autonomy in the career. Practice autonomy will need to include provisions for nurses to hire and supervise the auxiliary personnel who conduct nursing practice. A component of innovative practice models will need to include mechanisms of reimbursement for nursing services that will allow the nurse to move into higher salary levels of professional practice rather than being caught in the pattern of the low-wage worker.

Sparse examples of such innovative practice models exist in acute and long-term care. For example, nurses in the Twin Cities area have captured the critical care practitioners into a corporate model now contracting staff for intensive care services out to all hospitals in the area. Similar models exist in emergency services with emergency physicians, registered nurses, and life support personnel services provided to participating institutions. Another model emerging in long-term care is the teaching nursing home, where educators and practicing nurses form a team to design and test nursing practice interventions for debilitated chronically ill residents of nursing homes (Small & Walsh, 1988). In Chapter Twelve, Dison elaborates on innovative clinical models of care that have been created within hospitals.

The general public and health care providers other than nurses are often unaware of the various specialized roles nurses fill, the functions they perform, and the career options in areas other than clinical practice open to nurses. Addressing public stereotyped images of the nurse is a priority for the profession in order to provide long-term reversal of the disinterest in nursing by college freshmen (Green, 1987). Strengthening nursing's image has already begun through national and state professional leadership. Media campaigns and other ways of providing a more accurate portrait of the nurse are in place through the leadership of the American Nurses Association and affiliated state associations.

While the profession is changing in the workplace, nursing education programs will also need to take a serious look at the competence of their faculty and the relevance of the nursing curriculum within the context of the current patient care experience and the realities of the work setting. Meaningful relationships between educational institutions and hospitals and nursing homes are needed for retraining faculty and preparing nursing personnel who are able to function in revised systems of patient care delivery, including care of the patient with multisystem failure, long-term chronic maintenance care, and health improvement. Nursing has not advanced in areas of recruiting the nontraditional student or offering programs that allow for career progression. The allowance of transfer credit and special programs to recruit and retain the minority or older student are seldom found in nursing educational programs. Such mechanisms will be necessary to maximize the limited labor resources of the future.

The staffing of acute care hospitals, nursing homes, and home health agencies shows a lack of baccalaureate- and graduate-prepared nurses in roles requiring independent clinical decision-making, leadership, and management skills. The large proportions of diploma and associate degree technical nurses in positions requiring these advanced skills point to a limitation in the available supply of highly prepared nurses. Even in the nursing assistant positions, limited preparation for independent responsibilities, which continue to become more complex in nursing home and home health agencies, indicate that minimum requirements for these roles should include a high school diploma with additional formal nursing assistant training. Often, industries that compete for these personnel, the fast-food and hospitality industries, require, at the minimum, high school graduation for similar low-wage positions. Requisite skills for functioning in nursing homes include following increasingly complex procedures. Computer literacy, math skills, and the ability to read instructions are becoming more and more essential. Completion of the high school diploma is increasingly important for quality and efficiency in care.

Currently, nurses receive similar hourly wages despite the basic nursing education completed. There is little difference in the wages paid to nurses with diploma, associate degree, or baccalaureate education. Regardless of the kind of basic nursing preparation, licensure for entry into the practice world is the same. Once employed, the roles and functions of nurses prepared in the three educational programs will usually be the same. Advancement in terms of status and salary comes after attaining graduate education and specialization. The profession needs to assume leadership in either distinguishing the qualities of nurses from the three educational programs by providing for differing licensure provisions and clinical competencies or in accepting the notion that differentiation will occur at the time of specialization and earning graduate credentials. Whatever direction the profession chooses will need to be clarified to other health disciplines and to the general public.

The health care industries have important roles in dealing with the dilemma of assuring an adequate supply of registered nurses and other nursing personnel. Short-term incentives such as bounties for recruiting additional staff will have to be replaced with substantive change in the way nursing staff and other health personnel are recruited to deliver care in order to provide long-term solutions.

The public sector can play a part in the transformation of the role of the nurse to overcome the continued increased demand for nurses who are used in the traditional way. Creating priorities for baccalaureate and graduate education for nurses needed in leadership roles, particularly in long-term care, is one contribution public education policy is positioned to initiate. Public policy can also provide incentives to nursing education programs at all levels that provide avenues for the nontraditional student to access, transfer, and progress in education. Such incentives may be to provide special funding for nontraditional students and providing student loan and scholarship programs in partnership with the private sector. Already, some models for such programs are in place.

As the acute and long-term care industries reshape the roles and functions of nursing and other personnel, current statutory licensing language outlining the scope of practice of nursing and other health professionals will need to be redesigned to formalize the new images of health professionals. For example, in the acute care setting, there is much coordination and overlap among nursing personnel and other health disciplines such as respiratory therapy, pharmacy, and social work. In long-term care, nursing and social work provide essential elements in the care and placement decisions of debilitated and chronically ill persons who require comprehensive assessments and referral information. Reconfiguring these roles at a time when long-term care is expanding to meet the needs of an aging society will lessen the numbers of personnel needed and limit the duplication of services experienced by clients.

Our examination of federal projections for the future supply of nursing personnel demonstrated limited applicability to state nursing personnel needs because of identified shortcomings in the methodology of both historical trend- and criteria-based models used to project needs for future personnel (*Seventh Report to the President and Congress*, 1990). National and state projections of the need for nursing personnel must accurately reflect the unique demographic and services use patterns of the respective states as well as reflect the new use of the nurse in the redesigned health care system.

The public sector is a limited but important employer of nurses, particularly of public health nurses at the state level. Our findings of wages as much as 25% below the wages for nurses in comparable settings indicate that state career service salary structures need further examination. On the other hand, state benefits structures, particularly retirement benefits, partially balance the lower salary structures when compared with private sector benefits.

Throughout the health industries, we found limited pension benefits for nurses and nursing assistants. Although not examined in depth, we suspect from anecdotal information that, where pension benefits exist, the percentage of employer contribution to the program is lower than that in other industries and vesting times are extended. Reimbursement regulations may be a way of providing incentives for the health and long-term care industries to supply better pension benefits to their direct service workers. It is incongruous to conceive that the low-wage caretakers of today's elderly may well become tomorrow's impoverished elderly because of inadequate pension benefits associated with employment.

Reform through changes brought about by the profession, employers, and the public sector will create some resistance. In the past, attempts at change in nursing practice or education have stimulated resistance within the profession. Nurses who feel oppressed or do not affiliate with organized nursing can be the most vocal in a movement to restructure the profession and the workplace. Others will attempt to keep the roles of nursing and allied health professionals in the current tradition. Changes that may affect established practices in other disciplines, particularly for physicians, will be met with resistance from official association spokespersons. If threats to profits, or increased costs, are perceived as a result of change, then further resistance will occur from owners of hospitals and nursing homes. Such groups will need to understand the long-term benefits of altering traditional uses of nursing personnel to become part of the solution. For changes to occur, despite potential opposition from such sources, change is likely to be incremental rather than instantaneous.

Public policy and personnel programs will need to be examined closely in terms of how they affect the demand for and satisfaction of personnel in the health and long-term care systems. Dramatic changes in use and delivery of services have created the need for new skills and configurations of personnel. Lack of planning as these alterations have occurred within the system has caused a reactive environment in which increasing demand for traditional skills of the nurse has occurred. While the recent shortage of nursing personnel was more acute and widespread throughout the care delivery system than were previous episodes, there is much evidence that such shortages are in part influenced by industry personnel policies. Future expanding needs for services coupled with the realization that there are limited supplies of personnel predicted for the coming years are ample reasons for committing to a restructured system for nursing personnel practice.

References

Aiken, L. H. (1983). Nursing's future: Public policies, private actions. *American Journal of Nursing, 83*(10), 1440-1444.

Aiken, L. H. (1984). The nurse labor market. *Journal of Nursing Administration, 14,* 18-23.

Aiken, L. H. (1987). Breaking the shortage cycles. *American Journal of Nursing, 87,* 1616-1620.

Aiken, L. H. (1989). The hospital nursing shortage: A paradox of increasing supply and increasing vacancy rates. *Western Journal of Medicine, 151,* 87-92.

Aiken, L. H., Blendon, R. J., & Rogers, D. E. (1981). The shortage of hospital nurses: A new perspective. *American Journal of Nursing, 81,* 1612-1618.

Aiken, L. H., & Mullinix, C. F. (1987). The nurse shortage: Myth or reality? *New England Journal of Medicine, 317,* 641-646.

Allen, N. E., Nunley, J. C., & Scott-Warner, M. (1988). Recruitment and retention of Black students in baccalaureate nursing programs. *Journal of Nursing Education, 27*(3), 107-116.

American Association of Colleges of Nursing (AACN). (1987). *Reports on enrollments and graduations in baccalaureate and graduate programs in nursing, 1983-1987* (Institutional Data System series). Washington, DC: Author.

American Hospital Association (AHA). (1977-1987). *Hospital statistics.* Chicago: Author.

American Hospital Association (AHA). (1983-1987). National data network. In *AHA Annual Survey of Hospitals.* Chicago: Author.

American Hospital Association (AHA). (1988). *Hospital nursing personnel survey of 1988.* Chicago: Author.

American Nurses Association (ANA). (various years). *Facts about nursing.* Kansas City, MO: Author.

ANA fights cap on temporary agency fees. (1989). *The American Nurse, 21*(4), 13.

As the shortage takes its toll, some nurses are speaking up for better staffing. (1987). *American Journal of Nursing, 87,* 1694-1695.

Astin, A. W., Green, K. C., & Korn, W. S. (1987). *The American freshman: Twenty year trends, 1965-1985.* Los Angeles: University of California, Cooperative Institutional Research Program.

Astin, A. W., Green, K. C., & Korn, W. S. (1988). *The American freshman: National norms for fall, 1988.* Los Angeles: University of California, Cooperative Institutional Research Program.

Barhyte, D. Y. (1987). Levels of practice and retention of staff nurses. *Nursing Management, 18,* 70-72.

Barhyte, D. Y., Counte, M. D., & Christman, L. P. (1987). The effects of decentralization on nurses' job attendance behaviors. *Nursing Administration Quarterly, 11,* 37-46.

Beyers, M., Mullner, R., Byre, C. S., & Whitehead, S. F. (1983). Results of the Nursing Personnel Survey, Part 1: RN recruitment and orientation. *Journal of Nursing Administration, 13,* 34-37.

Bliesmer, M., & Eggenberger, A. (1989). Strategies for recruiting nursing students. *Nurse Educator, 14*(2), 17-20.

Boyer, C. M. (1979, March). The use of supplemental nurses: Why, where, how? *Journal of Nursing Administration,* pp. 56-60. (Reprinted in T. A. Duespohl, Ed., *Nursing in transition,* pp. 187-194; 1983, Rockville: Aspen)

Bracken, J., Clakin, J., Sanders, J., & Thesen, A. (1985). A strategy for adaptive staffing of hospitals under varying environmental conditions. *Health Care Management Review, 10,* 43-53.

Bridner, P. (1991). Solid gains behind, leaner times ahead. *American Journal of Nursing, 91,* 28-36.

BSN programs see new losses in enrollment. (1988). *American Journal of Nursing, 88*(4), 526, 542.

BSN rates are falling at a faster rate. (1987). *American Journal of Nursing, 87* (4), 529, 542.

Bureau of Economic and Business Research, University of Florida. (1980, 1987). *Florida statistical abstract.* Gainesville: Author.

Buzachero, V. V., & Parker, M. (1984). Sound recruiting with BMC soundsheets. *Personnel Administrator, 29,* 116-117.

Byerly, E. (1984). Estimates of the population of states: 1970 to 1983. In *Current population reports* (Series P-25, No. 957). Washington, DC: U.S. Bureau of the Census.

Carlson, S. M., & Cowart, M. E. (1988). *Shifts in supply and demand for nursing and other health care personnel in the 1980's: A review and evaluation of the literature.* Tallahassee: Florida State University, Institute on Aging.

Caron, C. (1989). *Survey report: Status of computer support in acute care hospitals in Florida.* Unpublished report, Baptist Hospital of Miami.

Center for the Promotion of Nursing. (1989). *Temporary staffing agencies: Solution or problem? A resource manual for hospitals.* Orlando: Florida Hospital Association Research and Education Foundation.

Clark, M. (1987, June 29). Nurses: Few and fatigued. *Newsweek,* pp. 59-60.

Cole, B. S., & Sizing, M. (1988). Cole nurse compensation. *Modern Healthcare, 18*(49), 24-47.

Coss, T. A. (1989). Nursing registries and economic efficiency. *Nursing Management, 20*(1), 50-51.

Cowart, M. E. (1982). *A comparison of attitudes, working conditions, and nursing practice of foreign nurse graduates and U.S. prepared nurse graduates in Florida.* Unpublished doctoral dissertation, Columbia University, School of Public Health.

Curran, C. R., & Minnick, A. (1989). *A model for improving retention of nurses in hospitals.* Chicago: Hospital Research and Education Trust.

Curran, C. R., Minnick, A., & Moss, J. (1987). Who needs nurses? *American Journal of Nursing, 87,* 444-447.

Curry, J. P., Wakefield, D. S., Price, J. L., Mueller, C. W., & McCloskey, J. C. (1985). Determinants of turnover among nursing department employees. *Research on Nursing and Health, 8,* 397-411.

Davidson, M. (1989, March). The temptation of temporary jobs. *USAID,* pp. 34, 36.

Davis, M. (1986). *Prisoners of the American dream: Politics and economy in the history of the U.S. working class.* London: New Left Books.

Deane, R. T., & Ro, K. K. (1979). *Comparative analysis of four manpower nursing requirements models* (Nurse Planning Information series). Hyattsville, MD: Health Resources Administration, Bureau of Health Professions.

Deets, C., & Froebe, D. J. (1984). Incentives for nurse employment. *Nursing Research, 33,* 242-246.

DeVries, R. G. (1986). The contest for control: Regulating new and expanding health occupations. *American Journal of Public Health, 76*(9), 1147-1150.

Downturn in aid puts new pressure on students. (1987). *American Journal of Nursing, 87*(4), 532.

Eastaugh, S. R. (1985). The impact of the Nurse Training Act on the supply of nurses, 1974-83. *Inquiry, 22,* 407-417.

Eggland, E. T. (1989). The role of supplemental nursing services. In T. F. Moore & E. A. Simendinger (Eds.), *Managing the nursing shortage: A guide to recruitment and retention.* Rockville, MD: Aspen.

Enrollments are rising again in BSN schools. (1990). *American Journal of Nursing, 90,* 106, 116-117.

Final report: The Legislative Study Commission on Nursing (1989, February). Raleigh, NC: Author.

Findlay, S., & Silberner, J. (1990, January 1). Costs and cures. *U.S. News and World Report, 107*(25), 68-69.

Flanagan, L. (1976). *One strong voice.* Kansas City, MO: American Nurses Association.

Flood, S. D., & Diers, D. (1988). Nurse staffing, patient outcome and cost. *Nursing Management, 19,* 34-43.

Flores, S. E. (1987). OR technical and professional staff: A study of California acute care hospitals. *AORN Journal, 45,* 97-108.

Florida Department of Health and Rehabilitative Services (DHRS). (1983). *Florida health manpower reports: Registered nurse survey.* Tallahassee: Author.

Florida Department of Health and Rehabilitative Services (DHRS). (1985). *Florida health manpower reports: Registered nurse survey.* Tallahassee: Author.

Florida Department of Health and Rehabilitative Services (DHRS). (1987). *Florida health manpower reports: Registered nurse survey.* Tallahassee: Author.

Florida Department of Health and Rehabilitative Services, Office of Comprehensive Health Planning. (1988). *Florida health manpower reports: Registered nurses, 1987.* Tallahassee: Author.

Florida Health Care Association and Association of Florida Homes for the Aged. (1987). *Nursing personnel shortage: A Florida nursing home problem of crisis proportions* (Mimeo). Tallahassee: Author.

Florida Hospital Cost Containment Board. (1985). *1983-84 annual report.* Tallahassee: Florida Department of Health and Rehabilitative Services.

Florida Hospital Cost Containment Board. (1986). *1985 annual report.* Tallahassee: Florida Department of Health and Rehabilitative Services.

Florida Hospital Cost Containment Board. (1987). *1986 annual report.* Tallahassee: Florida Department of Health and Rehabilitative Services.

Florida Health Care Cost Containment Board. (1988a). *1987 annual report.* Tallahassee: Florida Department of Health and Rehabilitative Services.

Florida Health Care Cost Containment Board. (1988b). *Nursing Home Reporting System annual report.* Tallahassee: Florida Department of Health and Rehabilitative Services.

Florida Health Care Cost Containment Board. (1989a). *Annual nursing home report.* Tallahassee: Florida Department of Health and Rehabilitative Services.

Florida Health Care Cost Containment Board. (1989b). *1988 annual report.* Tallahassee: Florida Department of Health and Rehabilitative Services.

Florida Hospital Association (FHA). (1985). *Nursing supply survey.* Orlando: Author.

Florida Hospital Association (FHA). (1987). *Nursing supply survey.* Orlando: Author.

Florida Hospital Association (FHA). (1988). *Nursing supply survey.* Orlando: Author.

Florida Hospital Association (FHA). (1989). *Nursing supply survey.* Orlando: Author.

Florida Hospital Association (FHA). (1990). *Nursing supply survey.* Orlando: Author.

Florida State Board of Nursing. (1987). *Annual report.* Tallahassee: Department of Professional Regulation.

Florida State Board of Nursing. (1988). *Annual report.* Jacksonville: Author.

Florida Statutes, Chapter 88-894, Section 3(1). (1988). Tallahassee: Secretary of States Office.

Ginzberg, E., Patray, J., Ostow, M., & Brann, E. A. (1982). Facing the facts and figures. *American Journal of Nursing, 87,* 1596-1600.

Gorman, C. (1988, March 14). Fed up, fearful, and frazzled. *Time,* pp. 77-78.

Gottfredson, L. S. (1981). Circumstances and compromise: A developmental theory of occupational aspirations. *Journal of Counseling Psychology, 28*(6), 545-579.

Grau, L., Chandler, B., Burton, B., & Kilditz, D. (1991). Institutional loyalty and job satisfaction among nursing aides in nursing homes. *Journal of Aging and Health, 3*(1), 47-65.

Green, K. C. (1987). What freshmen tell us: Excerpts from the transcript of the Nurses for the Future Conference. *American Journal of Nursing, 87*(2), 1610-1615.

Halford, G., Burkes, M., & Pryor, T. (1989, July). Measuring the impact of bedside terminals. *Nursing Management,* pp. 41-45.

Harrington, C. (1991). The nursing home industry: A structural analysis. In M. Minkler & C. L. Estes (Eds.), *Critical perspectives on aging: The political and moral economy of growing old* (pp. 153-164). New York: Baywood.

Hay, D. G. (1977). Health care services in 100 superior nursing homes. *Long Term Care and Health Services Administration, 300-313.*

Hay Group. (1988). *Nurse staffing, recruitment and retention in southeastern hospitals.* Atlanta, GA: Author.

Hinshaw, A. S., Smeltzer, C. H., & Atwood, J. R. (1987). Innovative strategies for nursing staff. *Journal of Nursing Administration, 17*(6), 8-16.

Holcomb, B. (1988, June). Nurses fight back. *Ms.*, pp. 72-78.

Holmes, P. (1987). Agency for change. *Nursing Times, 83*(18), 19-20.

Hospital-agency pacts said to be spreading like wildfire. (1989). *American Journal of Nursing, 89*(2), 277, 282.

Hospitals try new tactic to cut agency rates. (1989). *American Journal of Nursing, 89*(2), 276, 280, 282.

Huey, F. L., & Hartley, S. (1988). What keeps nurses in nursing: 3,500 nurses tell their stories. *American Journal of Nursing, 88*(2), 181-188.

In all weather, RNs battle for better staffing. (1988). *American Journal of Nursing, 88*, 371.

Irwin, R. (1977). *Guide for local area population projections* (Technical Paper 39). Washington, DC: U.S. Bureau of the Census.

Jensen, J. (1988, December 2). Nursing shortage fought on two fronts. *Modern Healthcare*, p. 48.

Jett, M. (1977). Use of temporary nursing personnel as a cost-control measure. *Hospital Topics, 55*(4), 48-50.

Johnson, W. L., & Vaughn, J. C. (1982). Supply and demand relations and the shortage of nurses. *Nursing and Health Care, 3*(9), 497-507.

Joint Commission on the Accreditation of Healthcare Organizations. (1990). *1991 accreditation manual for hospitals*. Oak Brook Terrace, IL: Author.

Kane, R. A., & Kane, R. L. (1987). *Long term care: Principles, programs, and policies.* New York: Springer.

Kearns, J. M. (1987). *The 1987 evaluation and update of the staffing criteria for the criteria-based model.* Washington, DC: U.S. Department of Health and Human Services.

Kehrer, B. H., Deiman, P. A., & Szapiro, N. (1984). The temporary nursing service RN. *Nursing Outlook, 32*(4), 212-217.

Kehrer, B. H., & Szapiro, N. (1984). Temporary nursing services: Size, scope, significance. *Medical Care, 22*(6), 573-582.

Korman, I. (1988, August 20). Eliminating the use of agency RNs: One approach. *Hospitals.*

Laird, D. D. (1983). Supplemental nursing agencies: A tool for combating the nursing shortage. *Health Care Management Review, 8*, 61-67.

Lewin, T. (1987, July 7). Sudden nurse shortage threatens hospital care. *New York Times*, pp. A1, A5.

Lipscomb, J., Toth, P. S., & Wurster, G. (1982). Nursing shortage threatens ward closure? An analysis of one medical center's response. *Hospital Health Services Administration, 27*, 18-25.

Long, B. (1984). Permanent relief for temporary woes. *RN, 47*(9), 21-23.

Manthey, M. (1988). Primary practice partners (a nurse extender system). *Nursing Management, 19*(3), 58-59.

Manthey, M. (1988-1989). *Consultation.* Minneapolis: Creative Nursing Management, Inc.

Marshall, V. W., & Longino, C. F., Jr. (1988). Older Canadians in Florida: The social networks of seasonal migrants. *Comprehensive Gerontology, 2*, 63-68.

Maryland crisis in nursing: Issues and recommendations. (1989). Annapolis, MD: Governor's Task Force to Study the Crisis in Nursing.

Massachusetts moves to limit agency charges but exempts pay rates for nursing personnel. (1989). *American Journal of Nursing, 89*(4), 552-553, 562, 564.

McCloskey, J. C. (1990). Two requirements for job contentment: Autonomy and social integration. *Image, 22,* 140-143.

McClure, M. L., et al. (1983). *Magnet hospitals: Attraction and retention of professional nurses.* Kansas City, MO: American Academy of Nursing.

McCulloch, E. (1989). *The Florida Department of Education Statewide Certified Nursing Assistant Workforce Study.* Leesburg, FL: Lake Sumter Community College.

McElreath, B. J. (1989). Why I'm an agency nurse. *American Journal of Nursing, 89*(5), 678-679.

McGillick, K. (1983). Modifying schedules makes jobs more satisfying. *Nursing Management, 14,* 53-56.

McLean, P. H. (1987). Reducing staff turnover: The preceptor connection. *Journal of Nursing Staff Development, 14,* 53-56.

Mershon, K. M. (1988, January-February). Nursing crisis: Demand for nurses outstrips supply as school enrollments drop rapidly. *Federation of American Health Systems Review,* pp. 21-24.

Mittan, J. B. (Ed.). (1989). *Florida health care atlas.* Tallahassee: Florida Office of Comprehensive Health Planning, Regulation and Health Facilities, Office of Aging and Adult Services, Department of Health and Rehabilitative Services.

Mohler, M. M., & Lessard, W. J. (1990, November). *Nursing staff in nursing homes: What it will take to remedy the insufficiency and what it will cost?* Presentation at the 43rd annual meeting of the Gerontological Society of America, Boston.

More patients, fewer nurses spelling trouble for emergency care services in many hospitals. (1987). *American Journal of Nursing, 87,* 1222-1223.

Motaz, C. J. (1988). Work satisfaction among hospital nurses. *Hospital and Health Services Administration, 33*(1), 57-74.

Munroe, D. J. (1990). The influence of registered nurse staffing on the quality of nursing home care. *Research in Nursing and Health, 13,* 263-270.

National Association of Health Care Recruiters (NAHCR). (1988). *NAHCR recruitment survey.* Springhouse, PA: Springhouse Corp.

National Center for Nursing Research. (1988). *Nursing resources and the delivery of patient care* (DHHS Publication No. 89-3008). Washington, DC: Government Printing Office.

National Commission on Nursing, Hospital Research and Educational Trust. (1981). *Initial report and preliminary recommendations.* Chicago: Author.

National Institute on Aging. (1987). *Personnel for health needs of the elderly through year 2020* (NIH Publication No. 87-2950). Bethesda, MD: Author.

National League for Nursing. (1986). *Nursing data review.* New York: NLN, Division of Public Policy and Research.

National League for Nursing. (1987). *Nursing data review.* New York: NLN, Division of Public Policy and Research.

Naylor, M. D., & Sherman, M. B. (1987). Wanted: The best and the brightest. *American Journal of Nursing, 87,* 1606-1605.

Neathawk, R. D., Dubuque, S. E., & Kronk, C. A. (1988). Nurses' evaluation of recruitment and retention. *Nursing Management, 19*, 38-45.

Nebraska Nurse Education Plan. (1989). (LP 890). Lincoln: Nursing Education Advisory Committee.

New federal commission will tackle the shortage. (1988). *American Journal of Nursing, 88*, 371, 378.

New Jersey State Nursing Shortage Study Commission. (1988). *Nursing Shortage Study Commission report to the governor.* Trenton, NJ: Author.

New salary wars promise solid gains this year: Hospitals are bidding up start and shift rates. (1988). *American Journal of Nursing, 88*(1), 113, 117, 120, 122.

Norhold, P. (1987). The nursing shortage: How bad is it? *Nursing, 17*(7), 28-36.

Nurses gained new economic ground this year. (1989). *American Journal of Nursing, 89*, 1674-1675, 1682.

Nursing home industry attacks temp agencies: Massachusetts will cap rates and set standards. (1988). *American Journal of Nursing 88*(11), 1563-1564, 1579.

O'Hare, W. P. (1976). Report on a multiple regression method for making population estimates. *Demography, 13*, 369-379.

Olson, S. K. (1983). The critical care nursing shortage: Are technicians the answer? *Dimensions of Critical Care Nursing, 2*, 229-302.

O'Reilly, M. E. (1987). Floating: A reality and a problem? *Focus on Critical Care, 14*, 60-61.

Pennsylvania RNs' salary goal is $30,000-$50,000 by 1990. (1988). *American Journal of Nursing, 88*(5), 737.

Postsecondary Education Planning Commission (PEPC). (1988). *Nursing education in Florida.* Tallahassee, FL: Department of Education.

Prescott, P. A., & Bowen, S. A. (1987). Controlling nursing turnover. *Nursing Management, 18*(60), 62-66.

Prescott, P. A., Dennis, K. E., Creasia, J. L., & Bowen, S. A. (1983). Supplemental nursing services: How and why are they used? *American Journal of Nursing, 83*, 554-557.

Prescott, P. A., Dennis, K. E., Creasia, J. L., & Bowen, S. A. (1985). Nursing shortage in transition. *Image, 17*(4), 127-133.

Price, J. L., & Mueller, C. W. (1981). *Professional turnover: The case of nurses.* New York: SP Medical and Scientific Books.

Rajecki, R. (1990, October). Climbing the nursing ladder: program boosts aides to LPNs. *Contemporary Long-Term Care, 52*, 112, 114.

Recruitment of foreign nurses grows as demand for services expands. (1982). *Hospitals, 56*(6), 49.

Regan, W. A. (1981). Supplemental staffing: Nursing personnel pools. *Regan Report Nursing Law, 22*(7), 2.

Regan, W. A. (1982). Hospital liability for agency nurses: Supplemental staffing. *Regan Report Nursing Law, 23*(9), 4.

Report of the Task Force on the Nursing Shortage. (1988). Harrisburg, PA: Subcommittee on Health (F. J. Pistellas, Chair).

Revicki, D. A., & May, H. J. (1989, Spring). Organizational characteristics, occupational stress, and mental health in nurses. *Behavioral Medicine*, pp. 30-35.

Richmond, D. (1987). Nursing: An endangered profession. *Modern Health Care, 16*(23), 32.

Roberts, M., Minnick, A., Ginsberg, E., & Curran, C. (1989). *What to do about the nursing shortage.* New York: Commonwealth Fund.

Robertson, M. (1987). Temporary staffing: A positive approach. *Nursing Management, 18*(7), 80, 82.

Rose, M. A. (1984). Factors affecting nurse supply and demand: An exploration. *Journal of Nursing Administration, 12,* 31-34.

Rosenfeld, P. (1988a). Nursing education in crisis: A look at recruitment and retention. *Nursing and Health Care, 9,* 283-286.

Rosenfeld, P. (1988b). Measuring student retention: A national analysis. *Nursing and Health Care, 9*(4), 199-202.

Salmond, S. W. (1985). Supporting staff through decentralization. *Nursing Economics, 3,* 295-300.

Salome, P. B. (1983). Monitor technician controversy. *Dimensions of Critical Care Nursing, 2,* 294-298.

Schmeling, W. H. (1990). Measures for image enhancement and recruitment approaches. In W. Serow & M. Cowart (Eds.), *Beyond shortage: Nursing personnel in Florida* (Vol. 4, pp. VI-1 to VI-47). Tallahassee: Florida Health Care Cost Containment Board.

Serow, W. J., & Cowart, M. E. (1990). *Beyond shortage: Professional nurses in Florida* (Vol. 2). Tallahassee: Florida Health Care Cost Containment Board.

Serow, W. J., Cowart, M. E., & Chen, Yen. (1990). Results of the nursing shortage survey: Hospitals, nursing homes, home health agencies and hospices. In W. J. Serow & M. E. Cowart (Eds.), *Beyond shortage: Nursing personnel in Florida* (Vol. 2, pp. IV-1 to IV-97). Tallahassee: Florida Health Care Cost Containment Board.

Serow, W. J., & Sly, D. F. (1988). Trends in the characteristics of the oldest-old: 1940 to 2020. *Journal of Aging Studies, 2,* 145-156.

Serow, W. J., Sly, D. F., & Wrigley, J. M. (1990). *Population aging in the United States.* New York: Greenwood.

Seventh report to the President and Congress on the status of health personnel in the United States. (1990). Washington, DC: Bureau of Health Professions, Health Resources and Services.

Shaheen, P. P. (1985). Staffing and scheduling: Reconcile practical means with the real goal. *Nursing Management, 16,* 64-72.

Sharp, J. Q. (1989). Nurse exchange: A creative approach to the nursing shortage. *Nursing Management, 20*(5), 92-94.

Sheridan, D. R., Bronstein, J. E., & Walker, D. D. (1982). Using registry nurses: Coping with cost and quality issues. *Journal of Nursing Administration, 12*(10), 26-34.

Shortell, S. M. (1990). *Effective hospital-physician relationships.* Ann Arbor, MI: Health Administration Press Perspectives.

Sixth report to the President and Congress on the status of health personnel. (1989). Washington, DC: Bureau of Health Professions, Health Resources and Services.

Small, N. R., & Walsh, M. B. (1988). *Teaching nursing homes: The nursing perspective.* Owings Mills, MD: National Health Publishing.

Speake, D. (1988). *Addendum to shifts in supply and demand for nursing and other health care personnel in the 1980's: A review and evaluation of the literature.* Tallahassee: Florida Hospital Cost Containment Board.

Speake, D. L. (1990). National trends and state comparisons. In W. Serow & M. Cowart (Eds.), *Beyond shortage: Nursing personnel in Florida* (Vol. 2, pp. II-1 to II-88). Tallahassee: Florida Health Care Cost Containment Board.

Speake, D. L., Cowart, M. E., & Schmeling, W. H. (1990a). Nursing recruitment and retention in Florida hospitals and nursing homes. In W. J. Serow & M. E. Cowart (Eds.), *Beyond shortage: Nursing personnel in Florida* (Vol. 4). Tallahassee: Florida Health Care Cost Containment Board.

Speake, D. L., Cowart, M. E., & Schmeling, W. H. (1990b). *Recruitment and retention of professional nurses.* Tallahassee: Florida State University, Institute on Aging.

Starr, P. (1982). *The social transformation of American medicine.* New York: Basic Books.

State board failure rate shoots up to 16.4%: Higher standards, lower "ability level" blamed. (1988). *American Journal of Nursing, 88*(4), 526, 542.

Statewide planning for nursing in Iowa. (1988). Des Moines: Iowa Board of Nursing.

Stern, M. (1982). Hospitals solve nursing shortage by arranging subsidized housing. *Hospitals, 56,* 42.

Stoops, R. (1983a). Nurse recruiting: Part I. *Personnel Journal, 62,* 272, 274.

Stoops, R. (1983b). Nurse recruiting: Part II. *Personnel Journal, 62,* 366, 369.

Stoops, R. (1983c). Nursing pool recruitment with a marketing approach. *Personnel Journal, 62,* 92, 95.

Stryker, R. (1982). The effect of managerial interventions on high personnel turnover in nursing homes. *Journal of Long Term Care Administration, 10,* 21-33.

Study sees RNs still gripped by pay compression. (1990). *American Journal of Nursing, 90,* 93, 112.

Styles, M. M. (1986). Two points to ponder about the shortage. *American Nurse, 18,* 5.

Styles, M. M., & Holzemer, W. L. (1986). Educational remapping for a responsible future. *Journal of Professional Nursing, 2,* 64-68.

Sullivan, E., & Decker, J. P. (1984). Solving the nursing shortage: Drawing nurses back to the hospital. *Health Care Supervisor, 2,* 79-86.

Tennessee plan for nursing for the year 2000. (1987). Nashville: Tennessee Commission on Nursing.

Texas nursing shortage: Situation and solutions. (1988). Austin: Texas Nurses Foundation.

Theisen, B. A., & Pelfrey, S. (1990). Using employee benefit plans to fight the nursing shortage. *JONA, 20*(9), 24-28.

Tonges, M. C. (1989). Redesigning hospital nursing practice: The professionally advanced care team (Pro-ACT™) model, Part 2. *Journal of Nursing Administration, 19*(8), 19-22.

Tucker, P. T. (1987). Recruiting nurses with an extern program. *Nursing Management, 18,* 90-91, 94.

U.S. Bureau of the Census. (1989). State population and household estimates with age, sex and components of change: 1981-88. In *Current population reports* (Series P-25, No. 1044). Washington, DC: Author.

U.S. Department of Health and Human Services (DHHS). (1982). *Nurse supply, distribution and requirements: Third report to the Congress.* Washington, DC: Author.

U.S. Department of Health and Human Services (DHHS). (1988). Secretary's Commission on Nursing final report (Vol. 1). Washington, DC: Author.

U.S. Department of Health and Human Services (DHHS). (1990). *The registered nurse population: Findings from the national sample survey of registered nurses, March 1988*. Washington, DC: Public Health Service, Bureau of Health Professions.

U.S. Department of Labor, Bureau of Labor Statistics. *Occupational outlook handbook* (Bulletin 2350; 1990-1991 ed.). (1990, April). Washington, DC: Author.

VerMeulen, M. (1988, June 12). What people earn. *Parade Magazine*, pp. 4-7.

Watson, P. (1990). The patient-focused model. In *Designing the future* (presentation). Lakeland, FL: Lakeland Medical Center.

Waxman, H. M., Carner, E. A., & Berkenstock, G. (1984). Job turnover and job satisfaction among nursing home aides. *The Gerontologist, 24*(5), 503-509.

Weisman, C. S., Alexander, C. S., & Chase, G. A. (1981). Determinants of hospital staff nurse turnover. *Medical Care, 194*, 431-443.

Wetrogan, S. I. (1988). Projections of the population of states, by age, sex, and race: 1988 to 2010. In *Current population reports* (Series P-25, No. 1017). Washington, DC: U.S. Bureau of the Census.

Williams, R. P. (1988). College freshmen aspiring to nursing careers: Trends from the 1960's to the 1980's. *Western Journal of Nursing Research, 10*(1), 94-97.

Wise, L. C. (1990). Tracking turnover. *Nursing Economics, 8*(1), 45-51.

Wood, J. B., & Estes, C. L. (1990). The impact of DRGs on community-based service providers: Implications for the elderly. *American Journal of Public Health, 80*(7), 840-843.

Zander, K. (1988). Nursing case management: Strategic management of cost and quality outcomes. *Journal of Nursing Administration, 18*(5), 23-30.

Index

National Center for Nursing Research, 239
National Commission on Nursing, 153
National Institute on Aging, 119
National League for Nursing, 7-8, 77
Naylor, M. D., 17, 25
Neathawk, R. D., 16
Nebraska, 41-44, 54-55
Nebraska Nurse Education Plan, 55
"New Federal Commission," 10
New Jersey, 41, 44, 46-47
New Jersey State Nursing Shortage
    Study Commission, 47
"New Salary Wars Promise," 88
New York, 216
Norhold, P., 4
North Carolina, 41-43, 56-57
Nott model, 21-22
Nunley, J. C., 84
"Nurses Gained New Economic
    Ground," 8
Nurse practice models. See Manage-
    ment
Nurse practice standards, 111-113
Nurse registries, 153
Nurse Training Act (P.L. 88-581), 2
Nursing assistant (certified). See Bene-
    fits; Educational programs; Ex-
    pense; Nursing personnel
    shortage; Recruitment; Reten-
    tion; Salaries; Turnover; Vacancy
"Nursing Home Industry," 157
Nursing homes. See Benefits; Character-
    istics; Employment; Expense;
    Health care industries; Labor
    force participation; Nursing per-
    sonnel shortage; Salaries; Staffing;
    Standards of practice; Temporary
    staff; Turnover; Vacancy
Nursing personnel shortage, xi, xiii, 1,
    3, 4, 31, 35, 36, 41, 219, 236, 239,
    242, 251, 257
  chronic, 1-2
  expenses, 113-114
  geographic distribution, 117
  nursing assistant (certified), 29, 121
  nursing home, 121-128
  position shortage, 3

registered nurse, 29
scheduling shortage, 3
seriousness, 36, 102-103, 111-112,
    121-122, 130, 136, 201-203, 239
size of institution, 117
strategies, 10, 13-26, 116
transient shortage, 3
Nurse specialties, 237
Nurse staffing, 12-13, 254
Nursing profession. See Professional
    nursing

O'Hare, W. P., 72
Olson, S. K., 21
O'Reilly, M. E., 20
Overtime expense. See Expense
Ownership. See Characteristics

Partners in Practice™, 220-222, 232
Pelfrey, S., 132
Pennsylvania, 41, 42, 60-61
"Pennsylvania RNs Salary Goal," 88
Personnel policies, 167-169
Philippines, 17
Postsecondary Education Planning
    Commission, 9
Population, 33-34
  older, xii, 33-34, 240
Poulin, M. A., 178, 220
Preceptorship. See Career advance-
    ment
Practice settings, xii, 43-44
Prescott, P. A., 3, 10-12, 18, 26, 117
Price, J. L., 117, 178
Pro-ACT™, 223
Professional:
  autonomy, 22, 25, 132, 230
  nursing, 237, 238-239, 252, 254, 256
  professionalization, 22
Public health nursing, 141-146
  See also Benefits; Turnover; Vacancy
Public:
  policy, 256
  sector, 255
  facilities. See Characteristics; Own-
    ership

About the Authors

James J. Bracher is the Executive Director of the Florida Health Care Cost Containment Board. As Executive Director, he has been central to the debate on such critical issues as indigent care, for-profit versus not-for-profit performance, and comparative health care information collection and dissemination. He has served as a consultant on health care costs, use, and development of health care benefit programs for business and nonprofit organizations. He has participated in numerous state, regional, and national seminars. Prior to his appointment in Florida in 1984, he was President of the Central Indiana Health Systems Agency, having served as Vice President for Administration from 1980 to 1982. He has also had experience in hospitals and the private sector. He is Chairman of the National Association of Health Data Organizations and a member of the National Association of Accountants. He received his M.B.A. and B.S. in accounting from Indiana University.

Susan M. Carlson is currently Assistant Professor of Sociology at the University of North Carolina at Charlotte, where she teaches courses in the sociology of aging, social problems, and quantitative methodology. Her recent research examines the impact of Equal Employment Opportunity laws on race/sex occupational and earnings inequality in the United States as well as cross-national differences in gender inequality in occupational outcomes between the United States and Sweden. In collaboration with Larry W. Isaac, she is analyzing historical processes of change in the Aid to Families with Dependent Children program and making cross-national comparisons of temporally varying wage regimes in the United States, Sweden, and other advanced capitalist nations. She is currently beginning a project that will examine temporal and spatial variation in intergenerational inequality produced by welfare state policies. She received her Ph.D. from Florida State University in 1987.

Yen Chen is currently Economic Analyst for the Office of Tax Research, Florida Department of Revenue. She received her Ph.D. from the FSU Department of Sociology with specialties in demography and economics. She has received special training in survey research and sampling as well as SPSS and SAS computer software. Her other degrees are the Master's of Demography from the University of California, Berkeley, and the Bachelor of Arts in English from the Peking Teachers College, Beijing. She was Research Associate in the Florida State University Institute on Aging and served as the data analyst throughout the study reported in this book.

Barbara J. Clark (M.P.H.) is Research Associate at the Florida Public Health Information Center at the College of Public Health, University of South Florida, Tampa. She was previously Project Coordinator for research studies funded by the National Institutes of Health and the Colgate Palmolive Company at the Universities of Florida and North Carolina at Chapel Hill. She has also evaluated Head Start programs for the U.S. Department of Health and Human Services.

Marie E. Cowart is Director of the Institute on Aging and Professor of Urban and Regional Planning at Florida State University, where she teaches graduate courses in the specialization on policy and planning in health and aging. She was co-principal investigator for the study reported in this volume. She is a Fellow of the American Academy of Nursing and of the Royal Society of Health and past President of the Florida Nurses Association. She served, as well, on the Task Force on Consumer Choice and Access in Health Care, the Florida Health Care Cost Containment Board, and the Task Force to Establish a Department of Elderly Affairs. Her research is in the areas of health beliefs and behaviors of older adults and supply and demand issues among nursing and other helping personnel. Her articles are found in *Nursing Outlook, Health Values, Research in Nursing and Health Care,* and *Journal of Family and Community Health.* She received the B.A. in nursing from the University of Florida, the M.A. in public health from Tulane University, and the Ph.D. in public health from Columbia University.

Charlotte C. Dison is Vice President of Patient Care Services at Baptist Hospital of Miami. Previously, she was Associate Administrator of Patient Care Services and Director of Nursing Services. She was also nursing supervisor at Beekman-Downtown Hospital in New York; staff nurse, operating room supervisor, and Assistant Director of Nursing Services at Appalachian Regional Hospital Association in Wise, Virginia; and staff and operating room nurse at Norton Community Hospital in Norton, Virginia. She holds the M.A. in Nursing Service Administration from Teachers College, Columbia University, and the B.S. from Florida State University. She has done postmaster's study at Nova University. She is certified in Advanced Administration from the American Nurses Association, received membership recognition in the American College of Health Care Executives, and was a Nurse Fellow with the Johnson and Johnson-Wharton Fellows Program in Management for Nurses at the University of Pennsylvania. She received the Florida Nurses Associ- ation Nurse Executive of the Year award in 1989 and the Florida Organization of Nurse Executives Nurse Executive of the Year award in 1990. In addition to holding faculty appointments and many leadership positions in professional associations, she served as a member of the Technical Advisory Panel for the study reported in this book.

Peter J. Levin is Dean, College of Public Health, and Professor of Health Policy and Management, University of South Florida in Tampa. He serves on the boards of the SSM Health Care Corporation and the University of South Florida Psychiatry Center. He consults for government and private organizations and has published on the topics of cost containment, health care system organization, managed care, workers compensation, and the management of hospitals in Japan. He is past Chairman of the Florida Hospital Cost Containment Board and co-chaired its Task Force on the Shortage of Nurses. He has served as Dean of the University of Oklahoma College of Public Health, Executive Director of Stanford University Hospital, and Associate Commissioner of the New York City Department of Health. He holds degrees from Harvard, Yale, and Johns Hopkins Universities and is a Fellow of the American College of Healthcare Executives.

Winifred H. Schmeling is Project Director for the *Strengthening Hospital Nursing: A Program to Improve Patient Care Implementation* grant at Tallahassee Memorial Regional Medical Center. The five-year, $1 million program is jointly funded by the Robert Wood Johnson Foundation and the Pew Charitable Trusts. Previously, she held a research position at the Florida State University Institute on Aging, which produced the study in this book. She was Executive Vice President of MGT of America, Inc., a Tallahassee-based management consulting firm and established the firm's health care consulting practice. She has consulted nationally for hospitals and other health care organizations as well as federal, state, and local governments in a number of areas including nurse recruitment and retention, survey and opinion research, hospital strategic planning, hospital marketing, health care market research, alternative delivery systems, and health care regulation. She received the B.A. in nursing from the University of Delaware and the M.A. and Ph.D. in health planning from Florida State University. Her experience includes clinical nursing; nursing education; nursing administration; state, regional, and community health planning; and health care consulting.

William J. Serow is Professor of Economics and Director, Center for the Study of Population, Florida State University in Tallahassee. He received his undergraduate degree from Boston College and his M.A. and Ph.D. degrees from Duke University. Prior to joining FSU's faculty in 1981, he served as Research Director of the Population Studies Center at the University of Virginia's Tayloe Murphy Institute. He has served as President of both the Southern Demographic and Southern Regional Science Associations, was a Fulbright Faculty Fellow in Demographic Economics at the Nether- lands Interuniversity Demographic Institute, and currently serves on the editorial boards of the *Journal of Gerontology-Social Sciences, Social Science Quarterly,* and *Review of Regional Studies.* He is the author of more than 70 papers published in professional journals and books as well as being editor or author of nine prior books.

Dianne L. Speake is Assistant State Public Health Nursing Director in Florida. She has held research positions at the Florida Health Care Cost Containment Board and at the Florida State University Institute on Aging as well as faculty positions at Florida State University and the University of Southern Mississippi. Her research interests include health promotion, gerontology, and health care delivery. Her articles on these topics have appeared in *Research in Nursing and Health Care, Health Values, Nursing Outlook,* and the *Journal of Community Health Nursing.* She received the B.A. and M.A. in nursing from the University of Mississippi, and the Ph.D. from the University of Texas at Austin.